Clinical Instruction in Lactation
Teaching the Next Generation

International Lactation Consultant Association (ILCA)

Developed by:

Phyllis Kombol, RN, MSN, IBCLC

Linda Kutner, BSN, IBCLC, FILCA

Jan Barger, RN, MA, IBCLC, FILCA

Clinical Instruction in Lactation:
Teaching the Next Generation

International Lactation Consultant Association

Praeclarus Press, LLC
2504 Sweetgum Lane
Amarillo, Texas 79124 USA
806-367-9950
www.PraeclarusPress.com

DISCLAIMER
The information contained in this publication is advisory only and is not intended to replace sound clinical judgment or individualized patient care. The author disclaims all warranties, whether expressed or implied, including any warranty as the quality, accuracy, safety, or suitability of this information for any particular purpose.

ISBN: 9781939807946

Table of Contents

Acknowledgements

No book is ever complete without acknowledging all the other people that helped make it happen.

We would like to thank Judi Lauwers, editor extraordinaire, who put as much time into the editing process as we did into the writing.

We are also grateful to the following people for their help in reviewing, commenting, and contributing to the text: Chantal Audoin, Gini Baker, Jessica Bilowitz, Gretta Blythe, Decalie Brown, Geraldine Cahill, Suzanne Campbell, Cindy Carter, Amal El Taweel, Denise Fisher, Adelina Garcia, Jacki Glover, Shakira Henderson, Hiroko Hongo, Maeve Howett, Vergie Hughes, Elly Krijen, Angela Love-Zaranka, Lisa Mandell, Mary Overfield, Carol Ryan, Bryna Sampey, Sue Saunders, Ann Seutens, and Meena Sobsamai.

Introduction

Women have received help from each other with breastfeeding for millennia. Beginning in the 1950s, help came primarily from mother-to-mother support groups. Today, it comes mostly from healthcare professionals. The lactation consultant profession was established in 1985, with the simultaneous founding of a professional organization, the International Lactation Consultant Association (ILCA), and the founding of the International Board of Lactation Consultant Examiners (IBLCE), which administers an international certification examination.

A role delineation study defines the elements of knowledge required for lactation consulting. Repeated periodically, it provides structure, referred to as a "blueprint," for the required knowledge for the profession and a list of competencies to be mastered in preparation for becoming an International Board Certified Lactation Consultant (IBCLC). Those competencies also form the basis of the accreditation standards defined by the Lactation Education Accreditation and Approval Review Committee (LEAARC). LEAARC, which is sponsored by ILCA and IBLCE, was formed in 2008 to guide education in the profession. Now, postsecondary academic programs may receive accreditation through the Commission on Accreditation of Allied Health Education Programs (CAAHEP).

The growth of the lactation consultant profession has paralleled that of other healthcare professions as they have become differentiated, along with the development of specifically defined educational preparation systems. Nurses, dietitians, and therapists (occupational, physical/physiotherapy, respiratory, and speech) have all experienced progress similar to what lactation consultants are now experiencing. For example, the first official nurses' training program, the Nightingale School for Nurses, opened in 1860. Imagine how the nursing profession looked in 1887, only 27 years into the life of that profession. More than 150 years later, nurses in the U.S. still struggle to define exactly what type of educational systems and preparation are best for the practice of professional nursing.

The education of professional nurses has moved from predominantly hospital-based diploma programs to the current degree programs offered through community colleges and universities. Programs of education for the nursing profession and other allied health professions are still evolving today, even after decades of growth. Lactation consulting is a very new addition to the allied healthcare professions. The ways by which lactation consultants are prepared for this profession are still very much a work in progress.

The goal of this text is to assist the clinical instructor in developing the type of internship that will best help individuals preparing for this profession to grow into competent and compassionate lactation consultants. The didactic and clinical experience individuals acquire in order to qualify to sit for the certification examination for IBCLCs are a beginning. However, the intent of a structured internship is to take an intern beyond the minimal clinical competency tested on the certification examination to produce a professional lactation consultant with supervised practical experience applying the knowledge and skills learned in coursework. The breadth of experience interns receive through a structured internship will not only maximize their potential to do well on the examination, but will also prepare the individual for the realities of providing lactation care. The IBCLC credential is considered to be the only internationally recognized certification and is the standard for the lactation consulting profession. Thus, use of the term lactation consultant describes someone with the IBCLC credential who is a fully prepared professional in the field of lactation consulting.

Students from any healthcare profession need to learn safe, professional practices in a supportive learning environment, with appropriate supervision and collaboration. Their instructors need to have certain experiences, attributes, and personality traits that will assist in creating a climate which facilitates the interns' growth. This text is designed to assist experienced lactation consultants in providing clinical instruction to prospective lactation consultants (interns). Structured internships prepare interns to practice as safe and competent lactation consultants and prepare them to take the IBLCE examination to become board certified. Parts of this text will be useful for prospective lactation consultant interns, as well, as they evaluate internship programs to determine what to expect or to design their own internships. The primary audience for this text, however, is the clinical instructor.

DEFINITIONS AND TERMINOLOGY

Because the vast majority of lactation consultants are female, feminine pronouns are used when referring to both the intern and the clinical instructor. This eliminates the cumbersome he/she or him/her. Definitions for other terminology used in the text are below.

BIRTHING SERVICES—Encompasses facilities which may be referred to as birth centers (with separate facilities and staff) or as departments within hospitals referred to as labor and delivery (L&D) units, mother-baby units/wards, nursery and postpartum wards.

CAAHEP—Commission on Accreditation of Allied Health Education Programs, which reviews and accredits post-secondary education programs. LEAARC is a review committee for CAAHEP for lactation programs.

CLINICAL INSTRUCTOR (CI)—Experienced IBCLC (recertified at least once) working with lactation as her primary focus, providing guidance and education to the lactation consultant intern in the clinical setting. Other sources may refer to this person as a mentor, preceptor, or trainer.

CODE—Refers to the International Code of Marketing of Breast-milk Substitutes and its subsequent World Health Assembly resolutions (WHO,

1981). According to the ILCA Standards of Practice (ILCA, 2006), all IBCLCs should adhere to the tenets and provisions of the Code as defined by the World Health Assembly.

CPC—Code of Professional Conduct for the IBCLC (IBLCE, 2011b).

DIDACTIC—Knowledge-based learning which may be delivered in a classroom or online through distance courses, webinars, or other electronic means.

DYAD—A mother and her baby (or a mother and her babies in the case of multiples).

IBCLC—International Board Certified Lactation Consultant who has met the credentialing requirements of the IBLCE.

IBLCE—International Board of Lactation Consultant Examiners, which designs and administers the credentialing process for IBCLCs.

ILCA—International Lactation Consultant Association, the professional organization of lactation consultants, regardless of certification status.

LACTATION CONSULTANT—Individual who is certified as an IBCLC and is qualified to practice safely and competently with breastfeeding mothers and babies.

LACTATION CONSULTANT INTERN—Student who has completed her basic lactation education and is in the process of obtaining clinical experience with mothers and babies under the supervision of at least one clinical instructor.

LACTATION INTERNSHIP—Period of time an intern spends in formalized training with an experienced clinical instructor.

LEAARC—Lactation Education Accreditation and Approval Review Committee, formed in 2008 to recognize educational programs and courses that meet the minimum standards of quality to prepare individuals to enter the lactation consultant profession. Name was changed in 2012 from AARC to LEAARC.

NICU—Neonatal Intensive Care Unit or SCN—Special Care Nursery— special units that care for preterm and sick babies.

WIC—Special Supplemental Nutrition Service for Women, Infants, and Children (USDA, 2011). As part of the U.S. Department of Agriculture (USDA), WIC provides nutrition education and supplemental food vouchers for eligible (low income and at nutritional risk) women and children. With a strong focus on breastfeeding promotion, support, and education, the WIC program employs IBCLCs and peer counselors, some of whom go on to become IBCLCs. The Canada Prenatal Nutrition Program (CPNP) is a similar program in Canada. Maternal and Child Health Service in Australia is a free service for all mothers and their infants, providing nurses qualified in early childhood care who staff well-baby clinics. Many of these nurses are also IBCLCs.

Chapter 1

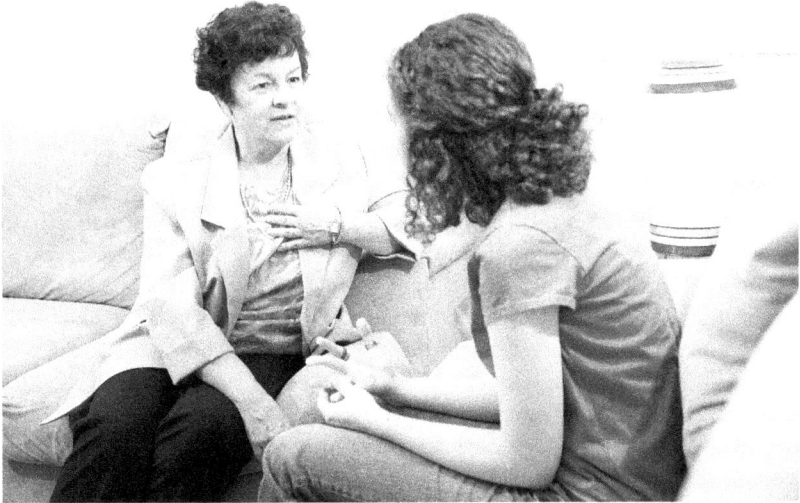

Standardizing Lactation Consultant Preparation

Lactation consulting is a relatively new allied health profession, with aspiring IBCLCs coming from a wide variety of backgrounds. In the early years, most IBCLCs in the U.S. emerged from the field of mother-to-mother support. Very soon, health professionals began to add lactation care to their primary professional roles. Today, the majority of IBCLCs in the U.S. and Canada are also nurses. Globally, IBCLCs come to the field from a wide variety of healthcare and allied health professions, with midwives predominant in many regions of the world.

Just as the backgrounds of entrants to the field are varied, so are the current methods by which they gain the necessary knowledge and skills. There are a variety of lactation courses available for different purposes. Some are ideal for people who are very new to the field, while others would be best for someone with a number of years of healthcare background. Some are self-paced, while others are quite structured within a specific time frame. The length of these courses ranges from a few hours to four years. Some courses are taught by independent educators. Others are taught in formal academic settings. Many lactation management courses that are designed as preparation for certification provide at least 45 hours of didactic instruction. In 2012 the International Board of Lactation Consultant Examiners (IBLCE) lactation education requirement increased from 45 hours to 90 hours for a candidates' lactation education. Many providers are increasing course length to meet this requirement. The increase to 90 hours is a step toward assuring that essential topics receive the attention they need.

Currently, many courses, especially those in the U.S., offer didactic instruction only and rely on graduates to arrange their own clinical instruction. In areas where a university or community college offers a program for lactation consultant education, the institution typically creates partnership arrangements for clinical placements. Organized clinical instruction specific to lactation is critical to the profession. It cannot be assumed, for example, that a healthcare professional with a background in maternal-child health has the necessary clinical background in lactation management to work as an IBCLC. A key certification issue is the quality and amount of didactic instruction and clinical/practical experience needed for an aspiring lactation consultant to become competent in performing clinical skills safely and to be able to make critical judgments and provide care to vulnerable populations. The impetus for this book is an attempt to explore ways that appropriate clinical education programs can and should be developed to accomplish these goals.

IBCLCs as Part of the Healthcare Team

To make positive contributions to the health and well-being of mothers and children, IBCLCs must be credible, recognized, and a valued part of mainstream healthcare. They work collaboratively with other healthcare providers on a multidisciplinary level to assure safe and effective, evidence-based care and best practices. Unfortunately, the formal education of most other healthcare providers includes little to no instruction in lactation physiology or principles of lactation management, education, and counseling. Thus, the practicing lactation consultant may be in an environment where lactation misinformation abounds.

IBCLCs Educate Other Healthcare Providers

Educating other healthcare providers is essential. IBCLCs should share, teach, recommend, and disseminate current information about evidence-based care practices. The process of dispelling myths, adjusting negative attitudes, and altering misguided beliefs is much more difficult than simply changing a knowledge base. Attitudes that view human milk feeding as unnecessary, difficult, dangerous, or hopelessly antiquated may seem almost insurmountable, making mere ignorance of the evidence seem to be a simple problem by comparison. This is part of what the U.S. Institute of Medicine defines as the "quality chasm" between evidence and practice (IOM, 2001), noting that not all healthcare practitioners have set aside personal preferences and anecdotal experience as rationale for care practices in favor of evidence-based care. Unfortunately, in many places, over 10 years later, this chasm still exists.

IBCLCs have a critical role and responsibility to aid other professionals in crossing that chasm.

OVERALL PREPARATION MUST BECOME STANDARDIZED

As members of the lactation consulting profession grapple with these issues, the need for standards in the preparation requirements of IBCLCs is increasingly apparent. Regardless of past requirements and practices, the education and clinical preparation of IBCLCs must reflect today's healthcare climate. There has been an explosion in the research base and available resources specific to lactation clinical practice, with several professional journals specific to the field of human lactation available internationally (Figure 1.1).

Figure 1.1. Professional Journals in Lactation

Breastfeeding Medicine (the official journal of the Academy of Breastfeeding Medicine) http://www.liebertpub.com/products/product.aspx?pid=173

Breastfeeding Review (the official journal of the Australian Breastfeeding Association) http://www.lrc.asn.au/bfreview.html

Clinical Lactation (the official journal of the United States Lactation Consultant Association) http://www.clinicallactation.org/

International Breastfeeding Journal (an open access, peer-reviewed online journal) http://www.internationalbreastfeedingjournal.com/

Journal of Human Lactation (the official journal of the International Lactation Consultant Association) http://jhl.sagepub.com/

Myriads of research and analysis of topics related to breastfeeding and lactation management appears in the journals of numerous other professions. Books and e-books about lactation care and management, once few in number, now fill huge displays at conferences. There are long lists of texts relevant to lactation on electronic media sites.

New mandates for the preparation of IBCLCs include standardization and formalizing in both didactic learning and practical application into consistent, evidence-based clinical skills. There are now sufficient numbers of experienced IBCLCs in many areas of the world who can guide those entering the profession.

While IBCLCs are increasing in number, only a small percentage of those practicing have the benefit of being surrounded by experienced colleagues with whom to collaborate in their day-to-day practice. Many IBCLCs practice in settings where they are the sole IBCLC. Thus, they make independent decisions, conclusions, and recommendations without the benefits of networking to confer with colleagues and share in the power of group brainstorming.

There are approximately 25,000 IBCLCs certified in the world.

TELEHEALTH TECHNOLOGY

Telehealth is a term describing the use of telecommunications technology to deliver health-related services. Global communication technologies make it possible to extend networking, teaching, and learning across distances to people in areas of the world where there is a low density of experienced professionals. Technology, such as voice over internet protocols (e.g., Skype), teleconferencing, videoconferencing, webinars, and similar strategies are effective tools for conferring with others who are geographically distant. In fact, these technologies are essential in many communities around the world, providing convenience, extended learning, and cooperative projects even in more densely populated areas.

Audio and video technology are embraced globally in various forms throughout the healthcare profession to provide in-home patient care. For example, the Health Resources and Services Administration in the U.S. Department of Health and Human Services has an Office for the Advancement of Telehealth (OAT) to promote the use of telehealth technologies for healthcare delivery, education, and health information services (HRSA, 2012). The use of interactive telehealth technology to assess and provide breastfeeding support in women's homes would be especially helpful in underserved rural and urban communities where women have no access to IBCLC care (Rojjanasrirat, Wambach, & Nelson, in press). It can be taken into the arena of assessment of clinical skills as well, with the instructor videoconferencing to supervise the intern's work. The real-time interaction made possible by telehealth technology broadens opportunities for lactation consultant students in remote areas. The technology is already in use for clinical assessment of skills in many areas of healthcare (RCGP, 2012; Turpin & Wheeler, 2011; Wagner, Keane, McLeod, & Bishop, 2008; Lindberg, Ohrling, & Christensson, 2007).

STANDARDIZED KNOWLEDGE BASE

Standardizing pre-certification lactation didactic education is an appropriate goal as the world moves further into the 21st century. It is quite possible that the lactation consultant profession will eventually mirror nursing, where a local community college or university includes a lactation curriculum and core health science courses necessary to award a degree in lactation sufficient to lead toward certification and practice as a competent IBCLC. Ideally, such a program will include the necessary clinical training in all the settings IBCLCs are employed, such as hospitals, doctors' offices, well-baby clinics, public health settings, private practices, and outpatient lactation clinics. The curriculum section of the Standards and Guidelines for Accreditation in Lactation Education follows this standard (CAAHEP, 2011). While the CAAHEP document is applicable internationally, there may be similar accreditation systems and curriculum guides in other regions of the world.

EDUCATION REQUIREMENTS FOR CERTIFICATION

Current requirements for certification include completion of eight general education subjects (Figure 1.2) and six continuing education topics (Figure

1.3). Some courses will combine two or more subjects and thus will meet more than one general education requirement (e.g., an Anatomy and Physiology course). In the U.S., students may be able to demonstrate mastery of college-level material by examination (IBLCE, 2011a). The College-Level Examination Program (CLEP) offered through the College Board offers exams to test knowledge acquired through general academic instruction, independent study, or extracurricular work (College Board, 2012). A similar program with examinations recommended for college credit by the American Council on Education (ACE) is the DANTES Subject Standardized Test (DSST) program (DSST, 2012). Both CLEP and DSST tests are administered throughout the year at colleges and universities in the United States and some other countries. For students who want to take these college courses in the U.S., accessibility may vary depending on previous educational background, educational system (university vs. private or community college), and whether the course is to be taken in person or electronically. In many countries, colleges and universities do not allow enrollment in individual courses and require full-year enrollment.

Aspiring lactation consultants with no health profession background are challenged by the length of time necessary to complete these requirements, as well as with obtaining practice hours and later employment. These individuals may consider pursuing preparation in a related profession, such as a practical/vocational nursing program in the U.S. In some countries, this would give the candidate licensure as a healthcare or allied health professional, meet all the educational requirements, facilitate access to hospitals and community facilities, and expand employment opportunities.

Figure 1.2. General Education Requirements

- Biology
- Human Anatomy
- Human Physiology
- Infant and Child Growth and Development
- Nutrition
- Psychology or Counseling or Communication Skills
- Introduction to Research
- Sociology or Cultural Sensitivity or Cultural Anthropology

Figure 1.3. Continuing Education Requirements

- Basic life support (cardiopulmonary resuscitation [CPR])
- Medical documentation
- Medical terminology
- Occupational safety, including security, for healthcare professionals
- Professional ethics for healthcare professionals
- Universal safety precautions and infection control

STANDARDIZED CLINICAL PREPARATION

The lack of consistency in the clinical background and education of those entering the field of lactation consultation calls for serious efforts at formalization and standardization in both clinical and didactic preparation. To be complete, clinical preparation will include psychomotor and behavioral skills and learning in the affective domain (attitudes and professional ethical role acquisition).

The three current pathways to certification differ widely in the number of hours of experience and degree of supervision required. Prospective certification candidates will find current requirements at the IBLCE website. The current three pathways are for:

> **Could core science courses be specific to lactation?**
>
> It would be fascinating to have access to a course such as "Biology of Lactation" or "Cultural Anthropology Related to Infant and Young Child Feeding," that would be specifically focused on the content and applications related to providing clinical care for breastfeeding families.

- On-the-job experience of healthcare professionals and mother-to-mother support counselors.

- Graduates from an academic program that integrates didactic and clinical instruction.

- Completion of a stand-alone, directly supervised clinical internship.

There is currently no requirement stating that clinical experience must occur after didactic learning or that it be integrated with didactic instruction. There are financial and professional risks involved when a candidate potentially accumulates hours of experience practicing incorrectly before acquiring necessary knowledge and theory that forms the basis for appropriate practice. Application of didactic knowledge to clinical situations near to the time of acquisition is preferable. Ideally, didactic and clinical instruction would be integrated throughout the intern's learning experience. In programs where the two components are taught independently, it is highly recommended that an aspiring lactation consultant complete all required didactic instruction before entering a clinical internship or acquiring the experience hours to qualify for the IBLCE exam.

KNOWLEDGE ALONE IS NOT SUFFICIENT FOR EFFECTIVE CLINICAL PRACTICE

Lactation consulting is not simply a "knowing" profession, but also a "doing" profession. An individual may have studied surgery, may have observed surgery, may have been the recipient of surgery, and may have even assisted in surgery. This does not translate into being capable of independently performing surgery. Competence develops faster when practice is supervised by a competent practitioner.

Historically throughout medical education, the "see one, do one, teach one" model was considered an effective and sufficient means for teaching competent clinical skills. However, achieving the level of expertise in a practice discipline involves subtler variations in skill acquisition. In her classic book *From Novice to Expert*, Patricia Benner applied the Dreyfus model of developing pilots' skills to the nursing profession. These include identifying novice, advanced beginner, competent, proficient, and expert levels (Benner, 1984). Table 1.1 presents Benner's Stages of Nursing Expertise adapted to lactation consulting, describing the progressive level of skills from novice to expert. It is expected that individuals beginning to make clinical judgments and recommendations for lactation management are also able to demonstrate the thinking skills Benner labels as "competent."

Table 1.1. Stages of Lactating Consulting Expertise

Stage 1: Novice	• May have no experience in lactation other than perhaps nursing her own children or seeing family or friends nurse their children. • Needs detailed instructions, rules, or "recipes" for everything she does; needs specific guidance and structure.
Stage 2: Advanced Beginner	• Is able to provide basic, respectful care. • Recognizes the important or meaningful aspects of a situation, but still sees situations as having various components, not as a whole. • Is beginning to have enough experiences that she can make accurate judgments in more common situations.
Stage 3: Competent	• May have some years of experience, though it may be limited in scope and breadth. • Has not yet been certified through IBLCE; may be preparing for certification. • Can organize and plan care to optimize both her and her client's time. • Is able to prioritize what she does; plans care so the more important issues are addressed first. • Coordinates multiple complex care demands.
Stage 4: Proficient	• Has three to five years of experience in a variety of settings. • Has recertified with IBLCE at least once. • Is able to visualize all the different stresses and issues a mother/family may be dealing with and adjust her plan of care accordingly. • Experience has shown her to avoid saying "never or always." • Understands that her clients are involved in complex situations, with lactation/breastfeeding being only one of the very many issues with which the mother is involved. • Is able to assist her clients in reaching their long term goals, rather than fixating on their short term goals. • Becomes proficient at multitasking.

Stage 5: Expert	• Has found what works for her, is flexible when complex situations arise, and is able to accomplish a great deal of work smoothly.
	• Is able to respond almost automatically, without having to consciously evaluate all the aspects of the situation.
	• May not even be completely aware of all the considerations that impact her practice decisions.
	• When she changes the way she practices, it is because it felt right to her, and she is able to support her judgments with other knowledge and experience that she has had.

Source: Adapted from Benner, 1984.

An intern will likely observe IBCLCs and other healthcare providers whose length of experience varies and who have a range of levels of expertise with specific skills. The intern will begin at the novice level, and as she progresses through the internship, she will begin to process information and experiences similar to the advanced beginner. By the end of the internship, she should be at the competent stage in most common lactation clinical situations. Many programs have recognized that relatively new lactation consultants, who may themselves be at the competent and proficient stages, provide fresh, concrete approaches to teaching newer interns and a willingness to share their newfound knowledge. While this is certainly a possibility for certain experiences, it is best to also have clinical instructors and program developers who have several years of lactation experience and experience with a wide range of situations or settings.

During clinical observations, the instructor can point out ways an interaction was individualized and how the thought processes led to the specific decisions that were made. The intern, as the novice, very likely will not be aware of these elements until they are pointed out. The intern with a bit more experience may function as an advanced beginner and may begin to formulate constants, such as, "We usually do it this way." An intern at the beginning of the competent stage will identify when a constant no longer applies, thus making adjustments and individualizing care. As an intern's proficiency develops, a practicing IBCLC, having more finely tuned skills, can incorporate multiple observations and decision-making opportunities simultaneously to customize the care she provides. This level of skill sets makes a great teacher of novices to experts.

Many times an expert IBCLC will respond naturally to subtleties or have developed intuition in certain situations. This "second sense" may make it difficult for her to step back and sort out the information absorbed from a clinical situation that made her choice of care "feel right" for a given circumstance. This is the challenge for an expert practitioner who is providing clinical instruction to the intern. How does one stop and remember everything that was seen, heard, and sensed that contributed to an automatic "knowing" of what to do next? Strong internship programs can be structured to take advantage of varying styles and skill sets by providing experienced IBCLCs with differing levels of experience for the intern.

Within the hierarchies of learning, one will recognize the difference between the cognitive domain, knowledge, and the skilled application of that knowledge, the psychomotor domain. Applying these domains, one finds there is a wide gap between passing a multiple-choice examination and effectively functioning as a provider of safe and effective care. Passing an examination does not equate to possessing the ability to think critically and quickly, to make decisions under pressure, and to communicate clearly. The affective domain, which includes internalized attitude and philosophy, must also be addressed, specifically including understanding of human rights issues and ethical decision making. Demonstrating skills effectively and explaining their rationale does not necessarily ensure that a practitioner views the mother-infant dyad holistically and recognizes the impact of extended family and other environmental influences. It may be more difficult for some practitioners to recognize the effect of their own interpersonal skills and responses on situations they encounter with mothers and their families. See Figure 1.4 for questions to consider when structuring clinical practice hours.

Figure 1.4. Questions for Planning Clinical Practice Hours

- Will the required hours be of a particular type of breastfeeding dyads with certain medical and/or physical conditions or simply acquiring a total number of hours?
- Will the required hours be within a specified time frame prior to the credentialing examination?
- Will the hours focus solely on the competencies necessary for an entry level IBCLC to practice safely?
- When will the hours occur in relationship to didactic instruction: before, after, or concurrently?
- Will expert level guidance be required or should an individual learn skills independently, discovering which techniques do and do not work within a caregiver role to mothers and babies?
- If accumulated hours are NOT supervised by an experienced IBCLC, what is the recourse when experiential conclusions and recommendations of the precertification learner are not evidence-based?
- What if there is no experienced IBCLC available to supervise a student? Could another practitioner be substituted?

SUPERVISED CLINICAL EXPERIENCE

Confusion concerning "supervised" clinical experience also needs to be addressed. Is it possible for the individual supervising the accumulation of clinical practice hours to not be a qualified IBCLC? Must this supervisor provide experienced guidance directly in the same space as the intern? Can the supervising IBCLC be distant yet available when needed or located at another site? The answer is "It depends!"

The degree of supervision needed depends on the intern's background and progression of skill development, role acquisition, and specific skills required in a given clinical situation. Rarely can a lactation consultant anticipate exactly what a particular clinical situation will entail before the interaction occurs. Skill development and progression may not be truly measurable in hours or even in number of experiences, since the variety of clinical experiences varies with the setting. However, it is possible and necessary to develop clearer recommendations and guidelines for acquiring clinical practice skills. An intern will need at least minimal familiarity with all the defined and essential lactation competencies and evidence to practice in a variety of settings. Furthermore, there needs to be a process for verifying the intern's thought processes behind the demonstration of a clinical skill.

ACQUISITION OF SKILLS

Assessing the acquisition of professional attitudes and philosophy in the affective domain is challenging and requires careful observation and listening on the part of the clinical instructor. A structured program, which includes written work, review conferences/seminar discussions, and other communication with the intern, enables the supervising clinical instructor to learn and evaluate the rationales and provide necessary guidance. This process allows the clinical instructor to gain insight into the intern's developing philosophy and self-perception as a professional, as well as to assist the intern in building her critical thinking skills.

Lactation consultancy continues to define itself as the profession evolves and as healthcare changes. Education needs to include the essential clinical practice skills and competencies critical and universal to the most basic and generic care (IBLCE, 2010). Every new practitioner of lactation consulting needs to receive guided practice in clinical elements within structured lactation clinical internships with qualified instructors.

SUMMARY

Although lactation consultancy is a new profession, it has made impressive strides in its brief existence. There is still much to be done to achieve educational consistency and to raise and maintain the skill levels of its practitioners. Standardizing the prerequisite didactic and clinical preparation of IBCLCs elevates each member of the profession to a credible, respected, and essential member of mainstream healthcare teams around the world.

The chapters that follow provide specific information about the qualifications of clinical instructors and interns, how to develop lactation internship programs, the internship experience, pathways toward IBCLC certification, and sample forms, protocols, and applications. This is an exciting time to be a lactation educator involved in the continuing growth of a fulfilling and interesting profession!

Chapter 2

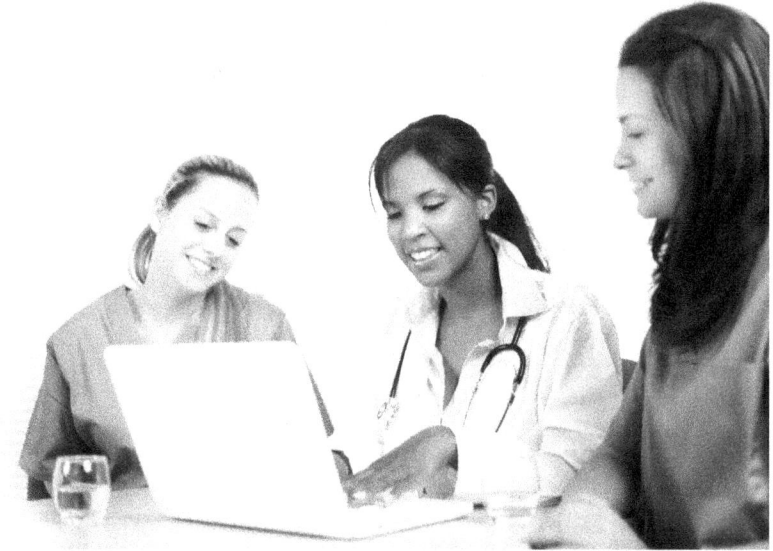

What Makes A Good Clinical Instructor?

It is easy to find individuals who want to be IBCLCs. In many parts of the world, there are programs in a variety of formats, styles, and locations that teach the essential didactic background of lactation consulting. What is missing are sufficient numbers of qualified individuals who will offer supervised clinical instruction for the preparation of IBCLCs.

Clinical instructors require a special skill set that enables them to guide new professionals in the application of knowledge and skills. Not all experienced IBCLCs want to serve as clinical instructors. Of those who wish to do so, not all will have the necessary teaching skills, experience, or professional and personal attributes that enable them to be effective clinical instructors. This chapter will explore what all good clinical instructors have in common and what can make them great.

DEFINITION OF A CLINICAL INSTRUCTOR

The words "mentor" and "preceptor" sometimes are used interchangeably to describe individuals who provide expertise and experience and act as a role model. Figure 2.1 demonstrates how the meaning of each differs subtly from one another and sets them apart from the definition of a clinical instructor. The term "clinical instructor" as used in this text describes the person who provides educational preparation to the aspiring lactation consultant.

Figure 2.1. Distinguishing Clinical Instructor from Other Terms

- **Clinical preceptors** are skilled practitioners who supervise novice practitioners in the clinical setting as they put into practice the skills they are learning. Precepting is often a formal part of an existing job, where the novice is currently employed and transitioning to a new position or is in orientation.
- **Mentors** typically serve as a role model and provide continuous guidance from novice student to qualified professional. Mentor relationships often go beyond the formal educational process and may last for years.
- **Clinical instructors** provide guidance and education to students in the clinical setting, within a formal, structured internship. The relationship between an intern and clinical instructor may evolve into a mentor/mentee relationship after the intern's formal clinical experience is completed.

FEASIBILITY OF BECOMING A CLINICAL INSTRUCTOR

An experienced IBCLC who wishes to become a clinical instructor must consider several practical issues to determine the feasibility of such a pursuit. A clinical internship requires a practice setting that will provide the experiences and instruction an intern needs. The instructor needs to be an effective educator, as well as having extensive experience with clinical situations. Interns need clinical instructors who can assess their knowledge and skills and nurture their professional development as clinical practitioners.

PRACTICE SETTING ADJUSTMENTS

In addition to having a desire to work with lactation consultant interns, a clinical instructor will critically assess the practice setting to optimize the intern's instruction. Restructuring can allow the additional time that is required for working with an intern. The instructor can incorporate the time needed to acquaint the intern with the clinical situation by including the intern in the chart review or in conversation with other caregivers before seeing a dyad. Time must be added into the consultation to allow the intern to be involved. The intern needs practice in providing direct care, which will require more time in the beginning when the intern is slower performing tasks and thinking through situations. After the consultation, more time needs to be allotted to debrief the intern on her impressions. Attention to these factors is essential before accepting lactation consultant interns, ensuring adequate time for learning and skill acquisition for competent practice as an IBCLC.

> **Consider...**
>
> You are the sole IBCLC in a medical facility that has 1500 deliveries per year, with a breastfeeding initiation rate of 80%. You typically see all the breastfeeding dyads in the maternity unit, NICU, medical/surgical and pediatric units.
>
> Will you have the necessary time and energy required to devote to an intern or is your reality just being able to care for the mothers and babies?

A large clinical practice is necessary to provide the clinical experiences an intern needs. This often requires collaboration with other IBCLCs and institutions where the intern can obtain clinical and counseling experiences the instructor cannot provide. Such networks may include experiences at birthing facilities, doctors' offices, public health clinics, NICUs, or outpatient lactation settings. Some clinical instructors accompany their interns to these off-site experiences, while others rely on individuals at these sites to supervise them. The instructor can assess the intern's level of engagement by reading and commenting on the written work and evaluations completed for these external experiences. This enables the clinical instructor to maintain her role as the primary instructor.

Professional networks among various practice settings provide great potential for collaboration, team teaching, and organizing joint lactation internships. An individual who has a private practice may find it much more difficult to provide experiences associated with birth practices, maternal-infant care during the first two hours post-birth, in-hospital care of well or sick breastfeeding infants, and hospital care of well or sick lactating women. Collaboration between clinical instructors in different settings and the intern's primary instructor expands a team teaching approach. Unless an intern's clinical instructor works in a large hospital complex associated with various doctors' offices and public health clinics, she will likely have a primary instructor and several site supervisors and other IBCLC instructors during her internship.

CLINICAL INSTRUCTOR QUALIFICATIONS

An effective clinical instructor should have basic understanding and skills of education processes, and, ideally, some experience teaching. In addition, a clinical instructor must have extensive experience over several years working directly with breastfeeding mothers and infants with a wide variety of clinical situations.

In 2012, the only qualification for a clinical instructor in Pathway 3 required by the International Board of Lactation Consultant Examiners (IBLCE) is being an IBCLC who has recertified at least one time (IBLCE, 2012a). It is expected that during the five years between initial certification and recertification, the IBCLC has refined her skills while working with breastfeeding mothers and babies. She would then have the necessary experience and insights to educate and train lactation consultant interns. However, there is no explicit requirement for verification that the time during that period was not spent working in a different field, raising a family, being a student, or being on medical disability. Working about 16 to 20 hours per week with breastfeeding dyads or more is likely to help the instructor refine her skills and maintain currency. Furthermore, actively caring for breastfeeding mothers and infants needs to have been her primary focus, rather than administrative responsibilities.

ESSENTIAL QUALITIES OF A CLINICAL INSTRUCTOR

Great instructors are life-long learners and love learning. They have the latest references and textbooks and are always ready to read another. Most have accumulated more journal articles than they can possibly read. Their level of experience and expertise allows them to consider new information objectively, and they are comfortable changing their practices and their perspectives when evidence dictates it. A good clinical instructor views the role of an IBCLC as a career and not simply a job. She belongs to her professional association, the International Lactation Consultant Association. She supports her profession by attending meetings and conferences, and participates in the local ILCA affiliate when available and other breastfeeding-related groups.

COGNITIVE AND PERSONAL CHARACTERISTICS

In the article, *What Makes a Great Clinical Instructor? Lessons Learned from the Literature*, Susan Bannister and colleagues (2010) define a clinical teacher as someone "who interacts with a student in the context of ongoing patient care." What sets them apart from other teachers is "the involvement in and teaching about a patient." Bannister states that teaching in the clinical area is complicated, "because the clinical instructor needs not only to diagnose and treat the client, but also diagnose and assess the intern's knowledge and skills." In the lactation consulting profession, the client consists of the mother-infant dyad and the clinical area is anywhere the breastfeeding mother and child receive care. This dual role of treating the mother and child while teaching and assessing the intern has been an ongoing subject for discussion among those who consider accepting interns. How does one provide good care for the breastfeeding dyad and, at the same time, focus on teaching the intern?

Bannister et al.'s 2010 article reviews literature published on effective clinical teaching between 1990 and 2006, citing 480 unique descriptors of good teaching. Figure 2.2 and Figure 2.3 describe some of the cognitive and noncognitive descriptions found in the literature (Irby, 1995; Sutkin, Wagner, Harris, & Schiffer, 2008; Masunaga & Hitchock, 2010; Buchel & Edwards, 2005; Goertzen, Stewart, & Weston, 2005; Gibson, 2009).

Figure 2.2. Cognitive Descriptors of a Good Clinical Instructor

- Is knowledgeable.
- Demonstrates clinical skills.
- Is well organized.
- Has excellent communication skills.
- Provides feedback.
- Explains concepts clearly.
- Sets goals and expectations.
- Provides direct supervision.

Figure 2.3. Noncognitive Descriptors of a Good Clinical Instructor

- Is enthusiastic.
- Is stimulating.
- Is encouraging.
- Creates a positive, supportive learning environment.
- Models the profession's characteristics.
- Focuses on the learner's needs.
- Interacts positively with students.
- Practices active listening.

Enthusiasm, first on Bannister et al.'s (2010) list of noncognitive attributes, is the most significant trait the intern will remember about her clinical instructor. An instructor who is enthusiastic about seeing mothers and infants, who displays a sincere desire to learn and teach, and whose eyes light up when she sees an interesting article is what makes an excellent clinical instructor. A clinical instructor who is eager to discuss interesting clinical cases with colleagues will be an effective teacher, one an intern will contact beyond the internship for continued encouragement, information, and mentoring. British poet Samuel Taylor Coleridge states, "Nothing is as contagious as enthusiasm" (Brainy Quote, 2012). The authors of this text agree with him wholeheartedly!

INTERPERSONAL SKILLS AND STRENGTHS

Effective communication skills are so essential that it is worth a look at Dale Carnegie's classic book, *How to Win Friends and Influence People* (Carnegie, 1936). Carnegie discusses how to be a leader who changes people without giving offense (and teaching is, by definition, an activity whose goal is to change someone). Figure 2.4 offers his suggestions about how to effect change without offending or arousing resentment. Figure 2.5 describes his advice on how to win others to your way of thinking. Other essential communication skills include the ability to organize your thoughts quickly to make a succinct response at a teachable moment, and analytical skills that assist in breaking complex tasks into manageable and understandable steps.

Figure 2.4. How to Change People without Giving Offense or Arousing Resentment

- Begin with praise and honest appreciation.
- Call attention to people's mistakes indirectly.
- Talk about your own mistakes before criticizing the other person.
- Ask questions instead of giving direct orders.
- Let the other person save face.
- Praise every improvement.
- Give the other person a fine reputation to live up to.
- Use encouragement. Make the fault seem easy to correct.
- Make the other person happy about doing what you suggest.

Source: Carnegie, 1936.

Figure 2.5. Twelve Ways to Win People to Your Way of Thinking

1. Avoid arguments.
2. Show respect for others' opinions.
3. If you're wrong, admit it quickly and emphatically.
4. Begin in a friendly way.
5. Start with questions to which the other person will answer yes.
6. Let the other person do a great deal of talking.
7. Let the other person feel the idea is his/hers.
8. Try honestly to see things from the other person's point of view.
9. Be sympathetic with the other person's ideas and desires.
10. Appeal to the nobler motives.
11. Dramatize your ideas.
12. Issue a challenge.

Source: Carnegie, 1936.

EXPERIENCE AND SELF-KNOWLEDGE

Having a background of teaching in diverse situations enables the instructor to recognize and meet the needs of interns with varied learning styles. Examples of teaching experience may be in formal classroom settings, professional conference presentations, presentations of didactic and/or clinical programs to other lactation consultants, providing in-service or webinar educational opportunities to other healthcare professionals, and teaching various kinds of breastfeeding classes for parents.

Awareness of the instructor's preferred teaching styles is also helpful. Teaching style can be tailored to particular circumstances and interns (Grasha, 1994). Table 2.1 adapts Grasha's work to apply it to instruction in the lactation consulting profession. A good clinical instructor will utilize the various styles and adapt them to the learning needs of each intern. The ability to use more than one teaching style is a sign of a good instructor.

Table 2.1 Teaching Styles

STYLE	DESCRIPTION	ADVANTAGE	DISADVANTAGE
Expert	The instructor processes the knowledge and expertise that she needs to instill in the intern, so the intern can function competently as a lactation consultant.	The instructor shares the information with the intern.	The instructor may overwhelm the intern and may use her "knowledge" to express her superiority to the intern. This process may fail to show the intern the underlying steps or thought processes that lead to the knowledge.

Style	Description	Advantage	Disadvantage
Formal Authority	Because of the instructor's knowledge base, she is viewed as an authority. In this mode the instructor follows "traditions" and standards of practice. She knows the rules, and supervises her interns very closely. She is concerned with the intern doing things in the correct and acceptable manner. This model provides the intern with the structure she needs in her early training period.	The instructor provides very clear expectations and requires that things be done in an acceptable manner.	An instructor who uses only this mode of teaching may become rigid and is not flexible in meeting different interns' needs and concerns.
Personal Model	The instructor believes in teaching by example. She wants the intern to observe what she is doing and to repeat back what she does.	This model emphasizes observing the instructor and doing return demonstrations exactly the way the instructor does them.	This model does not allow for doing things in different ways. The instructor may see her way as the only correct way of doing things. Some interns end up feeling they will never be good enough to be exactly like their instructor. This method may lead the intern to develop the philosophy that there is only one correct way of doing things.

STYLE	DESCRIPTION	ADVANTAGE	DISADVANTAGE
Facilitator	A personal relationship is established between instructor and intern. The instructor asks the intern questions to stimulate her thinking. She suggests options and helps the intern analyze them. She encourages the intern to be independent and to take responsibility for her actions.	The instructor is more flexible and able to focus on where the intern is with her learning. She is open to exploring options.	This method can be very time consuming. A new intern may find it intimidating and need more structure.
Delegator	The intern is encouraged to function autonomously, with the instructor nearby as a resource. This is an appropriate model when the intern has progressed to the level where she can provide safe, competent care to mothers and infants in most situations.	The instructor helps the intern learn to function independently.	The intern may not be ready to function in this capacity.

Source: Adapted from Grasha, 1994.

At the beginning of an internship, the instructor may mostly use formal authority and the personal model, progressing to using the facilitator style. As the intern advances through an internship, more collaborative styles, such as facilitator and delegator, may predominate. Taking a teaching styles survey, such as the online Grasha-Riechmann survey, may give instructors insight into their own typical dominant style and lead them to consider how adjustments may be made in certain circumstances (Grasha-Riechmann, 2012).

CLINICAL INSTRUCTOR AS ROLE MODEL

Conducting oneself professionally enables the clinical instructor to present herself as a reliable role model to interns (Figure 2.6). One element of professionalism is membership in her professional organization (ILCA). She should encourage interns to also become members. Another element is remaining up to date with advances in the field by pursuing continuing education through conferences, webinars, study modules, and other forms of self-improvement. Relevant to fostering the instructor's own professional development, currency demonstrates to the intern the need for lifelong learning and maintaining high-level skills. An average of fifteen hours of continuing education per year is required for maintaining certification as an IBCLC (IBLCE, 2012a).

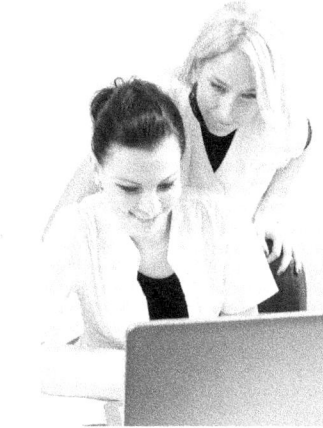

Figure 2.6. The clinical instructor serves as a role model to interns.

Maintaining high ethical standards is an indicator of the instructor's professionalism that sets the stage for the intern to develop a personal ethical code. The International Code of Marketing of Breast-milk Substitutes (WHO, 1981) and the IBLCE Code of Professional Conduct (IBLCE, 2011b) guide the IBCLC's ethical practice. A clinical instructor's adherence to the Code of Marketing requires not accepting direct funding from a nonCode compliant company or any other vendor that could have an influence on what or how she practices or what she teaches. Explaining to the intern the reasons for maintaining distance from such influence to the intern will be a challenge for the instructor since these concepts are frequently counter to what is commonly practiced in society, as well as in many work settings. Explanations and examples provide an opportunity for the clinical instructor who is familiar with the standards of both guiding documents to point out how these principles apply to numerous real-life situations that occur in clinical settings. Ensuring that interns become familiar with the Code of Professional Conduct will help them see how they are able to apply the principles in their daily professional encounters.

RESPONSIBILITIES OF A CLINICAL INSTRUCTOR

Much has been written by various authors, organizations, and healthcare specialists on what makes the best instructors and what their responsibilities should be. Adapted from the Millikin University description of a preceptor's roles and responsibilities, Figure 2.7 presents excellent points for a clinical instructor to consider (2006). It has been modified here using the terminology consistent with the role of clinical instructors in lactation consulting. Figure 2.8 describes important features of a clinical instructor's responsibilities that will ensure a successful experience for the intern.

Figure 2.7. Role of the Clinical Instructor in an Internship

- Demonstrate genuine interest in the lactation consultant intern.
- Be willing to commit time and expertise to help guide the intern – be accessible.
- Relate new concepts to the intern's prior learning when possible.
- Use good communication skills – actively listen, share, and respect the intern's input.
- Be flexible.
- Model professional practice and behaviors, and avoid restricting the intern to observing the instructor.
- Focus on the intern's strengths, while not overlooking their weaknesses.
- Promote independence as appropriate by using guiding strategies and problem solving techniques.
- Develop a trusting, open relationship.
- Help promote problem solving skills in the intern.
- Use reflection to help the intern learn from experiences.
- Use encouraging strategies.
- Be inclusive.
- Correct mistakes in a timely, supportive manner, focusing on remediation and how to avoid mistakes in the future.

Source: Milliken University, 2006.

Figure 2.8. Clinical Instructor Responsibilities to Ensure a Successful Experience

- Provide a thorough orientation for the intern and review workplace guidelines, especially those that will impact the intern's experience directly.
- Help the intern feel a sense of belonging in the workplace. Provide appropriate opportunities for the intern to participate in important agency functions, such as meetings and outreach events.
- Be aware of the intern's learning goals in order to provide guidance on how and when it will be appropriate to schedule certain experiences.
- Give honest, constructive feedback to the intern and other clinical instructors as needed.
- Meet with interns at frequent, regular intervals to provide feedback, evaluate progress, and resolve problems, both face-to-face and in writing.
- Remember that what may seem basic or easy for the clinical instructor may not be basic or simple to the lactation consultant intern.
- Pay attention early in the internship to determine the intern's learning style, as well as strengths and weaknesses. Appeal to the intern's strengths and address weaknesses constructively and with sensitivity.

Source: Millikin University, 2006.

NURTURING THE INTERN'S GROWTH

A good clinical instructor offers gentle guidance when she sees the intern floundering or going in the wrong direction. She is patient and willing to step back to allow the intern to work at her own pace. She is able to sense when an intern is ready to take on more responsibilities during interactions with mothers and babies. When a clinical instructor does not allow an intern to become involved in consultations, it is usually for one of four reasons, as described in Figure 2.9.

Figure 2.9. Reasons for Failing to Allow Interns to Participate

- The instructor feels the intern will slow her down and she doesn't have time for the intern.
- The instructor perceives the clients as "hers" and perceives involving the intern as losing control.
- The instructor feels unsure about her ability to teach the intern. She worries the intern will ask questions she cannot answer or that she may make a mistake that will reflect poorly on her.
- The intern is not competent and needs to be dismissed from the program.

INCLUSION OR EXCLUSION

Occasionally, a practicing IBCLC serving in a clinical instructor role may have a mother-infant dyad with whom there is an established relationship prior to the intern's entry into a clinical practice site. This dyad may have a sensitive issue, such as sexual abuse, and the intern's presence may compromise the care that can be given (Figure 2.10). It may also interfere with sensitive aspects of confidentially that have already been established between the IBCLC and the client. While there may be such times when an instructor must see a client privately, such occurrences are rare. Generally, when teaching interns, an instructor needs to relinquish the client relationship and include the intern in the interaction.

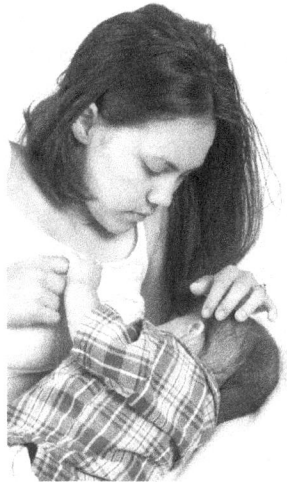

Figure 2.10. A mother's situation may dictate whether an intern is involved.

In an institutional setting, the consent the mother signs before seeing the IBCLC covers the intern being in the room and participating in the consultation. However, the mother deserves full disclosure about the intern's role and qualifications. An individual in private practice who accepts an intern may need to have the mother sign an additional consent form to include the mother's permission for the intern to be present and to examine her and her child. The intern will have signed a statement of confidentiality previously, regardless of where she is seeing mothers and children.

Most mothers are comfortable having the intern present for the consultation. Since the clinical instructor spends more time explaining things to the intern, the mother hears what is being said or sees what is being pointed out to the intern, and her learning is enhanced. Mothers will develop a relationship with the intern, as well as with the instructor. On occasion, when it is necessary to have the mother seen by another IBCLC, the mother may ask to have the intern present, even if the clinical instructor cannot be there. This is a wonderful indication of not only the ability of the instructor to involve the intern in the consults, but it shows that the intern has been accepted and valued as a part of the healthcare team.

THE INTERN AS PRIMARY FOCUS

When with an intern, the clinical instructor's primary focus should be working through the intern whenever possible to meet the needs of the breastfeeding dyad. At the same time, the instructor continues to have ultimate responsibility for the care given. The instructor continues to be involved with mothers and babies by supervising the intern who is taking the history, evaluating, assessing, and developing a plan of care. However, the instructor's primary role will be teaching the intern as these functions are performed, thereby nurturing the intern's growth. Thus, the clinical instructor does not trade off one aspect of her practice (responsibility to ensure appropriate care) to assume the role of instructor, but takes on the additional role of teaching simultaneously. Previously, satisfaction was gained solely through providing direct care to mothers and their children. Now there is the added satisfaction that comes through facilitating the growth, development, and achievements of the intern. This dual role may be difficult for an IBCLC who is not an experienced clinical instructor and whose primary focus has traditionally been her own clinical care provision and/or meeting expected productivity quotas in her facility.

PROFESSIONAL OBJECTIVITY AND PROFESSIONAL BOUNDARIES

The clinical instructor must maintain a professional relationship with the intern based on objectivity and high expectations. Addressing negative issues might be difficult and uncomfortable if an instructor and intern were friends or became personal friends during the internship. Setting structured rules, guidelines, and boundaries from the beginning of the internship may help with this. Maintaining professional boundaries allows for unbiased evaluation in the clinical and educational settings. Objectivity provides a basis for establishing a climate in which

Instructors must be careful to maintain professional boundaries with interns to:

- Not assume any form of financial responsibility for them.

- Not share leisure activities or personal time while the relationship is focused on being instructor and intern.

- Make sure their responsibilities and obligations are clearly stated and understood.

It can be difficult to maintain professional objectivity when compassion and personal feelings get in the way.

gossip, rude or crude jokes, and disparaging remarks about clients, doctors, IBCLCs, and staff are not be tolerated.

An important aspect of professional objectivity is to not expect more of an intern than she is capable of doing well. For example, the intern may exhibit confidence and excellent clinical skills assisting with early latch and positioning problems, yet need more support when confronted with a situation requiring more complex care, such as that required for a infant with a cleft lip and palate. Some interns (and IBCLCs) find their comfort with a certain level of breastfeeding problems, not wishing to participate in more complex issues. The clinical instructor is ultimately responsible for the care provided to breastfeeding mothers and children. An internship is a fine balance between expecting the intern to work to her full potential while providing safe care and challenging her to continue to learn.

SUMMARY

Why would an IBCLC have an interest in becoming a clinical instructor? Many IBCLCs will view this opportunity as a natural progression of professional practice. They may be motivated to share their expertise, perspectives, and wealth of experience and knowledge from many different clinical situations over the years. Experienced clinical instructors develop a recognized expertise and specialty in nurturing future professionals that attracts more students wishing to learn from them. The profession of lactation consultancy encourages and needs these women to share their expertise, keeping in mind that a teacher can make or break an intern's career. Selection of IBCLCs with education, qualifications, and the ability to enhance the intern's learning and love of the profession is crucial to the success of the internship program.

Chapter 3

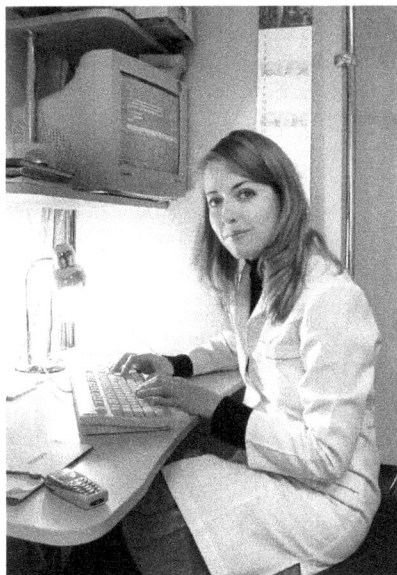

What Makes a Good Lactation Consultant Intern?

Prior to the advent of the lactation consultant profession, most organized assistance and support for breastfeeding was provided by mother-to-mother support groups. When the profession formally organized in 1985, volunteer counselors from these mother support organizations were predominant among those within the first several groups of candidates to take the IBCLC certification examination. Healthcare providers constituted another form of organized care. Globally, midwives typically have learned about breastfeeding during their formal education. Other providers, such as maternity nurses and doctors, relied to varying degrees on their personal experience when counseling and supporting mothers. Although evidence and practice have evolved, some continue to view the role of those assisting breastfeeding women through these early perspectives and have difficulty viewing the IBCLC as a profession separate from mother-to-mother support or healthcare roles.

SETTING REALISTIC EXPECTATIONS

When a clinical instructor hears the statement, "I want to be a lactation consultant," there are some initial open-ended questions that will help establish the inquirer's lactation knowledge base and where she is in the lactation consultancy entry process. Many who inquire may have little understanding of what professional lactation consulting as an IBCLC encompasses. Frequently, the enthusiastic inquirer (or a friend or family member) has had a positive experience with a practicing IBCLC while breastfeeding an infant. They may view being an IBCLC as an ideal way to help other mothers. Some may consider the profession as a pathway to make money and work a few hours a week, while providing time for family and other interests. Healthcare professionals licensed in other areas may consider the IBCLC credential as an added dimension to their other professional roles.

Becoming an IBCLC is more than liking breastfeeding and wanting to help mothers. It will require time, energy, education, and a financial investment for didactic preparation and clinical experience, which may discourage some. The reality of one's desire, circumstances, and the necessary requirements may not match their expectations. Understanding the nature of the profession and the focused knowledge and specific skill sets required will direct the aspirants to recognize the dedication and commitment inherent in the process of becoming a respected member of a healthcare team. Clear understanding of the profession and its expectations, combined with the prerequisites required, may take up to three years.

The clinical instructor has the perspective to help the applicant evaluate her current personal and professional life, including physical, psychological, financial, and mental resources. Consideration should be given to the financial and professional obligations necessary, so the applicant can determine whether she has the resources to meet those obligations. The instructor can help her determine if she possesses the time and resources in her life for this commitment and whether it can be combined with a full time job and/or family responsibilities.

DESIRED QUALITIES IN AN INTERN

The identification and selection of appropriate individuals for a lactation internship requires careful consideration and review. A clinical instructor who is aware of necessary precertification requirements and professional attributes should be directly involved in selecting potential interns. Developing appropriate candidates for the profession is a critical element in a clinical instructor's role. Successful professionals are products of designed internships that ensure interns will be successful in meeting their goal of obtaining the IBCLC credential. Figure 3.1 describes several professional attributes that are desired in an intern. Other important attributes relate specifically to best helping meet the specific needs of mothers and babies.

Figure 3.1. Desired Professional Attributes for an Intern

- Demonstrate a commitment to life-long learning.
- Demonstrate a respect for and commitment to lactation as an evolving professional field.
- Exhibit a positive demeanor.
- Be willing to consider her personal values, qualities, and skills.
- Possess effective communication skills in both verbal and written language.
- Possess effective coping skills needed during emotionally draining lactation consults.
- Possess critical thinking, logical problem solving, and good analytical skills.
- Demonstrate resilience in awkward situations.
- Be prepared to invest in caregiving relationships with clients.
- Understand concepts of family-centered care.
- Be able to explore ethical dilemmas.
- Recognize and admit to practice issues that require help and be willing to ask for that help.
- Expect to have a professional relationship, not a close friendship, with the instructor.
- Respond to instructor feedback in a structured and professional manner.
- Take complaints about the organization to the instructor, not to colleagues.
- Give positive and constructive feedback on how supervision is working out.
- Acquire and maintain professional liability insurance for work as an intern.

PASSION WITH PERSPECTIVE

The lactation consulting profession draws people who believe in the importance of breastfeeding and are passionate about it (Figure 3.2). Many have been members of breastfeeding support groups and/or have been involved in breastfeeding advocacy and public awareness activities, such as walks and sit-ins, to raise awareness and appreciation of the importance of breastfeeding. As a healthcare professional, however, passion is tempered with maturity and understanding about the dynamics it takes to be a strong advocate with colleagues who may not have this same passion or values.

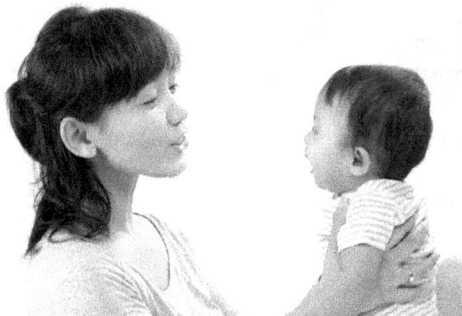

Figure 3.2. Compassion and a caring attitude are hallmarks of a good intern.

An intern will develop ways to cope with cultural, social, and commercial realities that do not reflect her perception of breastfeeding. She will also need to recognize that her personal beliefs cannot form the basis of her expectations of mothers. For example, an intern may be breastfeeding her three-year-old, yet does not expect the same of her clients. Similarly, she can experience delight when a teen mother breastfeeds for six weeks. When one is passionate about breastfeeding, often it can be difficult to put others' goals first. This is evident when a mother wishes to pump and feed from a bottle or when a mother says she wants to combine breastfeeding and formula feeding. The intern must develop perspective, so she does not overinvest in mothers who "might try" breastfeeding, while still providing ethical, effective, and compassionate care. When interviewing a prospective intern, it would be wise to interject these types of scenarios and ask what she would do, how she would feel, and how she would manage goals so different from her own.

BREASTFEEDING EXPERIENCE

It is not necessary that a prospective intern has breastfed her own children or that she has any children. It is necessary, however, that she be committed to promoting breastfeeding. That she has some experience with breastfeeding mothers and children broadens her compassion and empathy. Should she have children, her passion may stem from breastfeeding her own children, from struggling with feeding issues, or from regrets that she did not receive effective help. It may be that she was not able to reach her own breastfeeding goals. If she has no children, perhaps her experience has been through family members or friends who breastfed their children. Many individuals meet breastfeeding dyads in their work setting, and they may develop an interest in lactation and a commitment to helping mothers and children. Such familiarity with breastfeeding mothers and children is helpful before an intern begins her lactation education.

LOVE OF LEARNING

It is standard for academic texts to be updated at least every five years to ensure the most current information. The same is true for literature targeted to the general public. The need for constant updating of information in the case of breastfeeding and the lactation consulting profession is critical. The amount of information that is being published by related medical specialties exerting a major impact on breastfeeding and lactation is staggering. Regularly reading professional texts and articles ensures all in the profession an awareness of and a minimal acquaintance with new research. Thus, an appreciation of the value of life-long learning is a desirable attribute in a lactation intern.

OBSERVATION SKILLS

An ideal intern candidate is one who enjoys watching people and has the ability to interpret nonverbal cues. When watching people in large groups, such as an airport or shopping mall, she unconsciously reads and interprets the body language of others. The ability to read body language and verify the meaning of what is being observed is one of many hallmarks of a successful IBCLC. This attribute assists them in recognizing when a mother is so stressed she cannot absorb additional information. It alerts them to when a mother and/or infant who are overstimulated are shutting down. They will know that when a mother leans toward her with interest that she is receptive to more information.

Increasing an intern's ability to read body language is one of the most challenging aspects of a clinical instructor's role. The task becomes much easier if the intern is alert and sensitive to "people watching." The intern also needs to be aware of her own nonverbal messages, such as facial expression, body position, voice tone, speed of movement, and eye contact. She also needs sensitivity to the manner in which her nonverbal communications are perceived among different cultures. An intern's awareness of her interpersonal communication skills and challenges is important to her professional development.

Most literature available on reading body language focuses on the workplace or encourages the reader to exhibit positive body language when speaking to or directing others. Very few references illustrate or describe applications in a healthcare environment. Interns seeking resources on body language may use nonverbal communication sections in texts intended for counseling and nursing care professions or books from a local library (Andersen, 2004; Hagen, 2008; Kuhnke, 2007; Lambert, 2008; Lauwers and Swisher, 2011).

ENERGY AND BALANCE

A great deal of personal energy is required for helping new, stressed families. A vigorous store of enthusiasm and energy helps IBCLCs avoid emotional burnout. Without these resources, she may not fulfill her responsibilities in a professional manner. Assessing a prospective intern's personal energy level can be complicated. Discovering that a prospective intern is involved in numerous other activities may provide helpful insight in assessing her energy level and ability to balance and prioritize. Balancing enthusiasm and energy with the priorities and obligations of a profession are essential skills.

EDUCATIONAL BACKGROUND

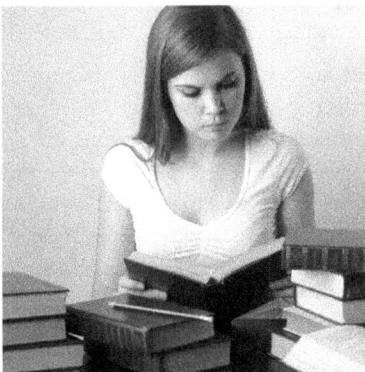

Figure 3.3. Becoming an IBCLC requires extensive learning and commitment.

Due to the diversity in educational backgrounds and precertification preparation within the lactation consulting field, there will be a wide range of diversity among interns. Some will express interest in the profession with little more than secondary education. Others will have completed college courses, and still others will have postsecondary degrees. Those with college experience are more likely to be acquainted with reading professional texts and articles, using a reference library, and doing an in-depth search of a topic on the internet (Figure 3.3).

They are more likely to write in a concise and professional manner, and to have the organizational skills to manage projects and meet deadlines. The attributes refined through the college experience will help the intern adapt to the requirements of an internship. Entering an internship at this level gives the intern an advantage and precludes the need for a clinical instructor to address these competencies remedially, while also teaching breastfeeding and lactation management skills.

FORMAL LACTATION PREREQUISITES

Current prerequisites for applying to take the International Board of Lactation Consultant Examiners (IBLCE) certification examination include general and lactation education and clinical experience. There are no parameters to the type of lactation education acquired. This may range from a comprehensive lactation management course to a series of continuing education activities, such as conferences and study modules. An individual clinical instructor or institution that accepts lactation interns may have requirements beyond the IBLCE prerequisites. Clinical instructors are encouraged to design formal, defined prerequisites for interns entering a clinical internship. Figure 3.4 presents questions to consider when establishing the prerequisites for clinical internships.

Figure 3.4. Prerequisites for Lactation Education

> • Will the internship require completion of a comprehensive lactation management course that prepares the intern for the clinical practice of caring for breastfeeding mothers and children prior to the internship?
>
> • Will the internship accept completion of a course focused on counseling and theory rather than one on clinical lactation management?
>
> • Will the internship accept completion of short, focused seminars, conferences, and study modules rather than a comprehensive lactation management course?
>
> • How many hours of didactic lactation education must be completed before entering the internship? Should all 90 hours of precertification lactation education be completed prior to entering the internship?

The timing of the intern's lactation precertification education is also a factor. IBLCE requires 90 hours of didactic lactation education within the five years immediately prior to sitting for the board examination. As continual changes occur in breastfeeding and lactation management, acquiring the most current evidence-based information and skills is essential to an intern's knowledge base. If there is a long lapse since an intern's initial lactation education, she may need to complete another current, evidence-based lactation management course prior to starting the clinical internship.

CRITICAL THINKING

Critical thinking needed for problem solving is one of the most important skills an intern will need to develop (Figure 3.5). The basics of critical thinking related to lactation care are more likely to have been taught in a course that is associated with skills development. A well-developed intern may also have had prior experience in practicing critical thinking skills in an educational or prior workplace setting. These interns can then continue to refine their problem-solving abilities throughout the internship. Clinical instructors need assurance that interns have a basic level of critical thinking that will assist them in assessing clinical situations throughout their internship.

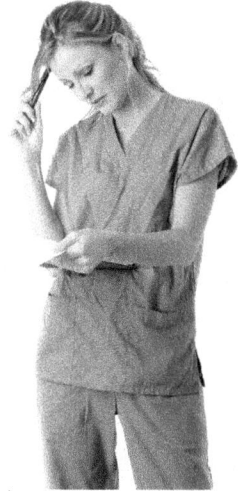

Figure 3.5 Critical thinking skills are essential to interns.

Clinical instructors can begin to assess an applicant's level of critical thinking by presenting hypothetical situations. For example, a mother has asked to see an IBCLC to address nipple pain. The instructor can ask what information the intern will need to assess the situation. Based on the applicant's responses, the instructor can then ask for the most probable causes for the soreness. Tailoring the scenario to lead toward a particular conclusion will help the instructor determine if the applicant is able to go beyond a routine recommendation that reflects this particular situation. Interns entering the program without formal instruction in critical thinking require more of the clinical instructor's time for teaching practical skills and their rationales. Table 3.1 presents an activity that will help a student learn the steps for critical thinking.

Table 3.1. Critical Thinking Activity

PROBLEM	Identify a problem a mother may have.	Nipple soreness
CAUSE	List all the reasons a mother may present with the problem.	
	Rank the causes according to those that are most likely to be seen.	
	Indicate the time period when each cause is most likely to occur: • First week postpartum • First few months after the birth • Months later	
HISTORY	Indicate a typical history for the problem.	
ASSESSMENT	Indicate the expected clinical findings following clinical and feeding assessment.	
PLAN OF CARE	Develop a plan of care for various cases based on the clinical findings.	

LEARNING METHOD

Lactation courses are available through both distance and classroom learning. It is the quality of education and not the presentation method of a completed lactation course that should be considered in acceptance into an internship. The desirable quality you will seek in an intern is the degree to which the student can participate actively in the learning process. Some learners prefer in-person discussions possible in a traditional classroom setting, citing the interactive dynamics of learning from and with fellow students. Virtual learning has progressed tremendously beyond instruction that simply presents information to recite at intervals throughout the course. Well-designed on-line courses can surpass classroom learning through active and interactive learning, including discussion groups. On-line courses also bring learning to the student at her convenience and remain available for repeated review. Many educational settings now incorporate multiple elements of in-person, multi-modal electronic access to audio/video recordings, as well as print and electronic media.

The availability of multiple learning modes can accommodate the various learning preferences of students. Instructors will recognize the diverse dynamics that certain courses provide for students with different backgrounds and learning styles (Kolb, 1984; Lawrence, 1991; McCarthy & McCarthy, 2005; McCarthy & O'Neill-Blackwell, 2007). In the final analysis, learning is what occurs inside the head of the learner, regardless of the styles or methods of education used.

CLINICAL EXPERIENCE

Candidates for IBLCE certification must acquire their clinical experiences within five years prior to taking the examination. The time it will take for an intern to complete all clinical experience hours required will be determined by the program design, the clinical instructor, and the intern. Interns spending 40 hours per work week in the clinical area may not allow time for the intern to analyze, process, and assimilate all of what was seen and done, particularly in the early part of the internship when they may be expected to write analyses of numerous experiences during the same week. However, being in the clinical area only a few hours a week extends the internship for a very long period of time. Recall the earlier assertion that a clinical instructor needs to work about 16 to 20 hours per week to progress and maintain skills. This same recommendation provides a good benchmark for an intern's expectation on the number of hours she will spend in the clinical area and the volume of clients she will need to see.

The amount of time the instructor and intern have available to work together will determine how the internship is structured. Time will be required for clinical days, written work, and research. Instructors who prefer not to have an intern with them every working hour may limit internships to around six hours per day. An intern who commutes long distances may need to work out a flexible design that accommodates a realistic schedule for herself and her instructors. The ultimate goal is to ensure that the intern is able to complete the internship in the timeframe required for qualifying to take the certification examination and to accomplish effective skill acquisition. Collaborating with multiple clinical instructors and alternate clinical sites to provide sufficient dyads and varieties of experiences help to achieve this goal.

Interns need to recognize that reading and studying will be required outside their commitment of weekly clinical hours. While working with mothers and babies, the intern will encounter many situations, diseases, and conditions not covered in their basic lactation management course. She will then need to research these issues in order to provide optimal care to the breastfeeding dyad. Understanding the expectation that outside work extends beyond the hours providing clinical care will help the intern plan realistically for the commitment of the internship and consider how it can be balanced with her other life responsibilities and commitments.

SUMMARY

Clinical instructors in formalized internship programs need to establish groundwork helpful to potential interns deciding if they wish to embrace lactation consulting as a career. This profession is not traditionally a job in which the employee works an eight-hour day, leaves the workplace, and does not think about it again until the next workday. A professional career as an IBCLC requires a willingness to spend a significant amount of offsite time in reading, researching, and preparing. It is expected that the clinical instructor view lactation consulting as a professional career and allot time in her life to keeping current. The clinical instructor is expected to prepare interns for a professional career in lactation and all the commitment it entails.

The quality of an internship is greatly influenced by the quality of the clinical instructors, as well as the qualities the intern brings to the experience. The most exceptional intern may fail to reach her potential if she is paired with a poorly qualified clinical instructor. A good clinical instructor will be expected to work equally well with either a well-prepared intern or one who is poorly prepared. By the end of the internship, the intern who learns the most from the program will be the one who puts the most into the internship, which may predict their ability to contribute to the lactation profession.

Chapter 4

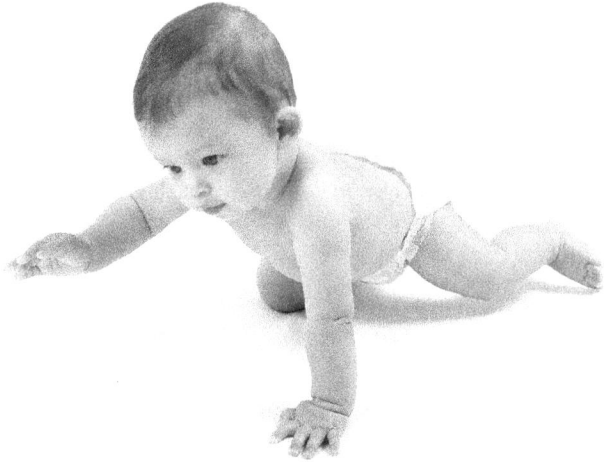

Developing an Internship Program

Providing interns with a solid foundation in lactation and breastfeeding management requires a wide variety of contributions from qualified clinical instructors. Creation of a clinical lactation internship program should occur in a systematic fashion that will ensure the necessary resources and support to sustain the program.

PREPARATIONS FOR AN INTERNSHIP PROGRAM

Planning an internship program begins with first taking an inventory of all the resources that can be committed to the program. This includes qualified staff, physical facilities, and the time that will be required for successful management of the program. Performing a detailed analysis of resources helps to determine the feasibility, design, and maintenance of a successful internship program. Figure 4.1 presents questions to consider during the planning process. After determining the program's feasibility, address administrative tasks regarding processing of applicants, finances, and conflict resolution. See Appendix 1 for a sample policy on maintenance of internship records. See Figure 4.2 for administrative issues to consider.

Figure 4.1. Determining the Feasibility of an Internship

1. Is there a need for such a program: why here and why now?

2. How many interns can you accommodate in your program at the same time?

3. Will you have enough dyads to support the establishment of an internship program? Review the number and types of breastfeeding dyads present in your institution or practice in the previous year. Consider the number of dyads you see each week compared with the number of hours and experiences the intern will need to have each week to finish the internship in a timely fashion.

4. Do you have the time and energy to develop and manage the program? How will you mesh it with your job, responsibilities, and professional development?

5. Do you have qualified colleagues to serve as clinical instructors? Do they have the time and energy to provide the wide variety of experiences? How will they mesh their job and responsibilities with the commitment to teach interns?

6. Do you have institutional support? Identify your support people before you get started, if for no other reason than to have others with whom you can discuss your ideas. Will your institution allow the necessary time during your workday to develop the program, teach interns, and manage the program? Remember, at first, it may take twice as long for clinical visits where you are teaching the intern.

7. What will you do when your practice is too busy to accommodate the time needed for teaching and supervising the intern? How can you provide meaningful learning experiences that do not require the clinical instructor's supervision or involvement?

Figure 4.2. Administrative Considerations

1. Will you and all of your clinical instructors meet and discuss each application or will you create an admission team who reviews the applications, interviews applicants, and makes sure all the prerequisites are met before accepting the intern into the program?

2. Who will maintain educational records, write letters of reference, and communicate with IBLCE concerning interns who plan to sit for the certification examination?

3. Who will manage financial issues, such as billing, disbursements to the proper accounts, and refunds for interns who leave the program (e.g., withdrawal or dismissal)?

4. How will you manage dismissing an intern from your program? What legal advice and paperwork will you need before being faced with this?

5. How will you handle conflicts that arise between instructors, between instructors and administration, between instructors and the interns, or between clients and the intern? Who will mediate such conflicts?

ACQUIRING INTERNS

Due to the challenges of finding a structured clinical experience, an internship program may have no problem acquiring interns. Potential interns may struggle to locate programs where supervised clinical experience is available. Finding didactic education is less challenging because of the variety of courses now available; finding sites to acquire the required clinical experience is the hard part. ILCA's Clinical Instruction Directory lists available clinical sites. Registering sites on this directory provides valuable information to prospective interns, describing specific aspects of various programs (ILCA, 2012a).

Directors of lactation education courses are eager to refer students to sites to acquire clinical experience and are tremendous resources for clinical internship programs. Periodically, send multiple copies of flyers about your program; do not expect course directors to print them for their students. You can also reach potential interns by adding your internship program to business cards to distribute at conferences, workshops, and affiliate meetings, along with flyers that describe the program.

ENROLLMENT OF PARTICIPANTS IN A LACTATION INTERNSHIP PROGRAM

There are a number of issues to be considered concerning the process of enrolling participants into a lactation internship program. These will be defined as the program is designed: what will the admission requirements include, how will the program be marketed, how will interested individuals indicate their interest in enrollment, how will applicants be screened and selected, and how will expectations of the program be expressed. Figure 4.3 describes the sequence of events in the enrollment process.

Figure 4.3. Sequence of Enrollment Events

1. Prospective intern decides to explore doing an internship and makes initial contact in person, by phone, or via website to review the program description and have questions answered.

2. Eligibility is determined with confirmation that all prerequisites have been completed.

3. Prospective intern determines which course will best meet her needs, completes the application, and submits it to the internship program (see Appendix 2 for samples of the application form, application, and enrollment checklists).

4. Program administrator reviews the application and associated documentation (e.g., transcripts, course records, references, credentials, and essay) and refers the applicant to clinical instructors to arrange an interview.

5. An interview takes place. The intern is approved and receives a letter stating that acceptance is pending completion of enrollment requirements, which may include tuition deposit, background check, drug screen, health/immunization update, proof of current certification in cardiopulmonary resuscitation, verification of malpractice insurance and other requirements regarding safety, privacy, etc. The intern also receives a participant handbook of policies.

6. Preclinical screening is completed and the intern is scheduled to receive a facility orientation, parking permit, and identity badge. If the internship requires written work before clinical hours are scheduled, it will be submitted and reviewed at this time.

7. A departmental and internship orientation is scheduled with the clinical instructors.

8. The internship schedule is established and the internship commences, along with evaluations as defined in the policies. Time logs, skills checklists, and written work/feedback are used throughout. As completion of the internship nears, final evaluations of the intern, the clinical instructor(s), and the program are requested.

9. A letter or certificate of completion is awarded after all materials are submitted.

ADMISSION REQUIREMENTS

Having a written description for prospective interns or a website with the prerequisites for program admission and completion will avoid misunderstandings. Figure 4.4 identifies elements to consider in determining your admission policies. Admission materials must clearly state that completion of the internship program does not guarantee employment with you, your institution, or any other institution. After having read the prerequisites and disclaimers, a prospective intern can complete an application (see Appendix 1 for an example). An essay explaining why she wants to be a lactation consultant could be included in the application process. The quality of the essay may help in determining an applicant's acceptability. After accepting the application, you can schedule an interview allowing sufficient time for application review and to contact references.

Figure 4.4. Admission Policy Considerations

- What basic lactation education will be accepted? IBLCE requires a minimum of 90 hours of lactation education. Will this be achieved through a comprehensive lactation management course or various forms of continuing education?

- Must interns complete the college and continuing education courses required by IBLCE for individuals who are not healthcare professionals (see www.IBLCE.org) prior to admission? Most experienced clinical instructors would recommend this. If not completed prior to admission, will they be able to complete this requirement during the internship?

- How can the intern demonstrate understanding of how to access, evaluate, and use research and principles of evidence-based care?

- How can the intern be asked to demonstrate the ability to communicate as a professional both verbally and in writing?

- Will the program or facility accept nonhealthcare applicants? If so, how will the program be adapted for different backgrounds?

- Will the program or facility accept only licensed healthcare professionals? These candidates will be familiar with the healthcare industry, medical terminology, informed consent, comfort in the clinical setting, and discrete handling of private healthcare information. They will probably fit in easily with the staff at clinical sites.

- What healthcare screening and background checks are required for your institution? Requirements typically include current immunizations and a health screening, drug screen, and a criminal background check. There may be fees involved.

- Most healthcare facilities require organizational orientation programs and other requirements which all new employees (interns included) must complete. How are these scheduled? Note that time to meet these requirements cannot be applied to clinical experience hours toward certification.
- The intern needs some form of professional liability insurance throughout the internship. In the U.S., individual professional liability insurance is available to lactation consultants and interns. An intern who is a licensed healthcare professional may choose to maintain that licensure and insurance, or seek lactation-specific insurance. In other countries interns may receive such coverage through the hospital or academic institution.

THE INTERVIEW PROCESS

Everyone interviewing the candidate should be thoroughly familiar with the application and noted areas that need to be explored. Ensure that the interview team gains sufficient insights through the initial inquiry, application, and interview process to assess a candidate's ability to write and speak professionally. Identify areas the applicant may find challenging, if accepted, so the intern is prepared to meet those challenges. Figure 4.5 lists possible interview questions.

Figure 4.5. Interview Questions

- Why do you want to be a lactation consultant?
- What do you think is the role and impact of an IBCLC?
- How do you anticipate fitting the internship into your life?
- What kind of breastfeeding conditions and situations have you encountered? How did you handle them?
- What do you feel will be the most difficult part of the internship? Why?

POLICIES AND EXPECTATIONS

The interview is an appropriate opportunity to explain fully the expectations of both the clinical instructor and the intern. Internship policies and expectations can be incorporated into a participant handbook (see the table of contents for a handbook in Appendix 3). Program expectations of interns and of the amount of work the program will encompass should be made explicit. A full description of program requirements, including both clinical and written work, is best presented prior to the interview. Reviewing a course syllabus (see the sample syllabus in Appendix 3) that describes activities and expectations offers the intern the opportunity to ask questions and discern her ability to fulfill the requirements. Figure 4.6 provides some guidelines for what to cover in the interview.

Figure 4.6. Interview Guidelines

> - Be explicit about the detail requirement of written work, when it will be due, and any follow-up required.
> - Encourage the prospective intern to discuss her goals for the internship and after certification as an IBCLC.
> - Review the internship schedule.
> - Provide a written plan for payment.

PAYMENT POLICY

Payment guidelines for whether and how internship fees are charged will vary by institution and region of the world. Figure 4.7 presents various options for charging fees. When a clinical instructor works for a healthcare institution, the intern will pay the institution. It is the responsibility of the clinical instructor to determine how she will manage her obligations both to her institution and to the internship program during her workday. Discuss with the institution whether review of any required written material will be accomplished on the instructor's off duty time or as part of the workday. Occasionally, an intern may pay her clinical instructor directly, with clinical experiences being conducted on the instructor's days off. This arrangement is not desirable nor professional, as the instructor is being paid by both her institution and the intern. This could be perceived as a potential conflict of interest.

Figure 4.7. Intern Fee Options

> - Charging an application fee.
> - Charging for blocks of hours.
> - Charging a daily fee for each day the intern is with a clinical instructor.
> - Charging a flat fee to cover the entire internship. Typically, the fee is divided and paid at predetermined points during the program. The total flat fee may be required before beginning the program.

Some clinical instructors in private practice contract with their interns to provide a specified number of hours of clinical experience, and in return, the intern works for free for a set period of time as an assistant to the instructor. This compensation by in-kind service is not currently a common approach, but may work for some individuals. For decades, the U.S. military has trained physicians and advance practice nurses with the condition of repayment in years of service. Such arrangements must be specified in writing in a memorandum of understanding or a contract to avoid misunderstandings. It may also be advisable to specify alternatives or consequences for breach of contract.

A written refund policy outlining the program's obligations that is made available to the intern prior to commencement will prevent later misunderstandings should an intern withdraw prior to or partway through the internship. If the intern withdraws 30 days prior to beginning the program, a refund of the entire amount less a small administration fee may be reasonable. If the intern withdraws a quarter or half way through her internship, a percentage of the fee could be refunded. Most institutions do not permit refund of any fees after the halfway mark. These details may be different for the intern in a program where she obtains all of her clinical experience hours than it will be for the intern with a clinical instructor for a shorter period of time.

ACCEPTING THE INTERN

Some internship programs accept new interns only at certain times of year for organizational planning or to match academic calendars. This should be specified in the program description. The applicant should be told how and when acceptance will be communicated and what the next steps will be. Reviewing the program's expectations again after the intern has been accepted affords an opportunity to reaffirm her commitment or to withdraw if she cannot fulfill the requirements. If she doubts her ability to complete the internship, it is best to make that decision before the program begins. Upon acceptance, the intern will need to present evidence of liability insurance and a copy of her current license if she is a healthcare professional. See Appendix 2 for sample applications and enrollment checklists.

PLANNING A PERSONALIZED INTERNSHIP

It may be difficult to accept all interns for a defined period of time. Depending on the intern's background, she may need more or less of certain experiences. Some individuals seek an internship despite having the necessary hours to qualify for the IBLCE examination, as they recognize they lack exposure in certain areas. These individuals may be with the program for a shorter period of time than an individual who needs experiences in all areas of lactation clinical competencies (see Appendix 4).

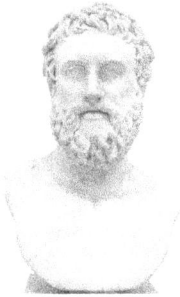

Consider...

"It is impossible to begin to learn that which one thinks one already knows" (Greek sage and Stoic philosopher, Epictetus—AD 55–AD 135).

Key point: Interns must be willing to accept that they don't already know everything.

A well-designed internship program offers both partial and full internships and personalizes each internship experience to a particular intern. It is commonly found that interns overestimate what they think they already know. Clearly communicating the applicant's level of preparedness is essential when designing a program that best meets her needs. The issue of preparedness needs to be presented in such a way that the intern recognizes it as a constructive assessment of her needs rather than personal criticism or an attempt to negotiate more hours than she needs. Ultimately, it is the intern's decision on how many hours she can afford to spend in an internship program. Having well-defined objectives and outcome measures, such as specific skills checklists or quantities of experiences, will provide structure for both the instructor and the intern to measure progress against the necessary lists of skills and competencies for lactation consultant practice.

To ensure the intern acquires necessary clinical hours, the clinical instructor should periodically review the hours already documented, so there is agreement regarding the number of hours accomplished. This will avoid having the intern's application to sit for the certification examination rejected because she failed to acquire an adequate number of clinical hours. It also assures the intern of receiving the clinical experience necessary to practice effectively at the end of the internship. Clinical instructors want to know they are producing and recommending well-prepared interns to both the IBCLE and to prospective employers.

Detailed questioning during the application, interview, and acceptance process helps both the clinical instructor and intern design a program that provides the number of clinical hours and particular clinical settings and experiences the intern will need. This should be incorporated into a signed agreement between the intern and the clinical instructor. A clause can be added stating that should the clinical instructor or intern determine that more clinical hours are needed in order to reach clinical competency, the agreement can be amended at any time during the internship to reflect this.

Interns are responsible for maintaining accurate records of their experiences and hours, with supervision by the clinical instructor or individual responsible for student academic records. Reviewing and signing them weekly or monthly helps to maintain currency and identify what remains to be accomplished (see the Clinical Experience Log in Appendix 4). Accurate record keeping and effective tracking of the intern's progression of skills is essential to the success of the internship program.

DESIGNING THE INTERNSHIP PROGRAM

The internship program should provide skilled clinical instructors whose combined supervision of the intern will produce a competent clinician who qualifies to sit for the certification examination. Careful selection of qualified instructors ensures coverage of the required clinical experiences, as well as the nonclinical activities that round out the internship program.

The appendix contains numerous forms to assist in the design of an internship, including both clinical and nonclinical learning activities. The worksheet, "Nuts and Bolts of Planning Clinical Experiences in Lactation," (USLCA webinar, March 20, 2012) in Appendix 1 is a starting point for foundations in program development. No matter how many details are put in place, something will always arise that was not anticipated. Also included in the appendix is a sample program developed between a large community hospital and a community college (Appendix 2), program applications (Appendix 2), evaluations (Appendix 5), and check lists (Appendix 4). These forms may be adapted for use in designing a program and completing details for each component.

ARRANGING FOR CLINICAL INSTRUCTORS

Acquiring applicants usually is not a difficult challenge; qualified clinical instructors are much harder to locate. An intern seeking clinical instructors may have limited selection choices. The intern will spend a significant amount of time with and money for her clinical instructor. She will want to make sure it is the best choice for her needs. Careful selection of qualified and skilled instructors to assist with clinical experiences will increase the likelihood of a quality learning experience for the intern. See Appendix 1 for a sample clinical instructor application and a sample contract between the intern and clinical instructor. The intern may want to meet with the instructors before starting the program or during the interview to assure this compatibility.

WORKING WITH MULTIPLE INSTRUCTORS

Working with multiple instructors provides interns the opportunity to see how different clinicians approach similar situations. Flexibility in clinical practice is often difficult for an intern or even a new IBCLC to accommodate. With more experience it becomes clear that there may be more than one correct way to approach a problem, depending on the situation. It is natural for an intern to prefer one instructor over another or to learn more from some than from others. Lessons learned in diversity and problem solving naturally evolve while working with multiple instructors and are very valuable aspects of the intern's education.

When a program relies on multiple clinical instructors, a process for communication between instructors regarding an intern's skills progression will be required. This avoids unnecessary duplication and facilitates agreement among instructors on expectations for the intern. Regular, open communication between primary instructors, interns, and various external instructors is essential to the success of an internship program.

TIME MANAGEMENT

A clinical instructor's consultation with a mother and child in a hospital setting will take longer to complete when an intern is present. Scheduling of additional IBCLCs, if available, allows for the extra time. The same applies when a private consultation is scheduled by appointment. These longer appointments can be noted in an appointment book and on the intern's schedule to avoid unnecessary waiting for clients.

Avoid closely scheduled consecutive consultations to allow time between clients to discuss the assessment, evaluation, and plan of care. It is during this debriefing that the intern has the opportunity to explain her rationale and to ask questions. Discussion between the instructor and intern after a consultation is one of the most important opportunities for teaching and learning. Do not underestimate the power of this time for rapid learning!

CREATING CLINICAL EXPERIENCES

Interns need to understand when they will simply observe the instructor and when they will participate in direct care during consultations. It is acceptable to spend a day observing at a special clinic or public health service. However, the intern should not spend an entire week restricted to simply observing others conducting outpatient consultations. This is not productive time. If the intern is quite inexperienced, she may be asked to weigh the baby or participate in the clinical setting in other small ways. Some interns need more time than others to be comfortable with progressive skills. Additionally, individual clinical instructors may need time to ease into trusting the intern with the care for which they feel ultimately responsible.

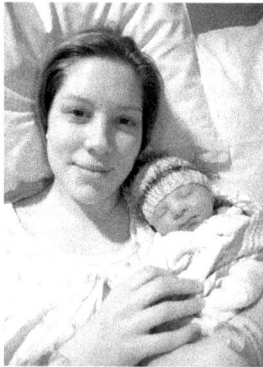

Figure 4.8. Interns need experience in a variety of clinical settings.

In recording the clinical experience hours, the intern and clinical instructor need to remember that hours that apply toward IBLCE Pathway 3 requirements are supervised clinical hours in which the intern is actually caring for the mother and child. However, this will require some judgment, since encounters often include both observation and direct care. While observation hours may be included in clinical internships for other IBLCE pathways, the idea of clinical experiences for an intern requires the intern to actually experience giving care.

An internship program that provides a wide variety of experiences will best prepare the intern for the varied situations she will encounter as an IBCLC (Figure 4.8). Experiences in the prenatal period, the public health setting, pediatrics, and breastfeeding support groups will be obtained within the community. Those acquired in the hospital include birth settings, the early postpartum period, special care nursery, and any other areas in the hospital providing care for breastfeeding mothers and children. Outpatient lactation clinic exposure, experience with private practice lactation consulting, and the business aspects of a practice complete the intern's clinical experience. See Appendix 1 for a sample memorandum of understanding for a clinical site.

A curriculum for a clinical internship should be based on the skills and abilities that the intern needs to achieve to become a competent IBCLC. Examples of activities and experiences that may be encountered in the various clinical sites can be found in *Clinical Experience in Lactation: A Blueprint for Internship, 3rd edition* by Kutner and Barger (2010). Many clinical instructors and interns in the U.S. use this resource. There may be similar resources in other regions of the world. Appendix 4 presents competencies that are based on that text and the IBLCE Pathway 3. The competencies are broken down into their essential components to assist the clinical instructor in helping the intern achieve mastery of the skills.

PRENATAL PERIOD

Exposure to breastfeeding information, family dynamics and support, and healthcare provider information during the prenatal period may influence a woman's intent and desire to breastfeed and eventually her feeding choice. Having an intern assist with teaching prenatal breastfeeding classes and assisting in prenatal consultations facilitates this positive influence on a woman and provides valuable experience for the intern. Spending time in an obstetric practice, midwifery clinic, or infertility clinic provides opportunities for discussing breastfeeding with women who plan to have babies. The instructor may arrange for the intern to follow a mother throughout her course of pregnancy, birth, and early breastfeeding, which provides insights into the new mother's needs during this important time. The intern can also use this time to research positive and negative interventions that may affect a woman's choice and ability to breastfeed.

PUBLIC HEALTH CLINIC

Many countries have high numbers of low-income families with young children. Over 50% of all mothers and children in the United States are low income and eligible for Special Supplemental Nutrition Service for Women, Infants, and Children (WIC) (USDA, 2011). Interns benefit greatly from exposure to the operation of public health clinics, some of which may specifically serve low-income breastfeeding mothers and children. WIC in the United States, Canada Prenatal Nutrition Program (CPNP) in Canada, and Maternal and Child Health Service in Australia are examples of public health programs where interns can acquire clinical experience. A large percentage of the clients an intern will experience in clinical practice will very likely be served by such clinics. Spending a day or two in a public health clinic will help interns understand the degree of education and support mothers receive during their clinic visits. Many U.S. public health clinics employ IBCLCs. An intern who plans to work in this setting may schedule more of her clinical experience hours in this setting.

PEDIATRIC CARE

In many locations, new mothers are usually advised to have their infants examined by a healthcare provider within a short time after discharge from their place of birth. Interns gain valuable insights by spending several days in a setting that cares for healthy newborns or participating in well-infant home-visit services. They can see what new mothers experience at this first newborn visit, as well as during visits with older babies. Encourage interns to observe the breastfeeding information, materials, and support offered to mothers, while evaluating both positive and negative aspects.

SUPPORT GROUPS

Where communities have mother-to-mother groups, the focus of the group is to support breastfeeding mothers and babies. While attending these meetings, interns can carefully observe and recognize the advice and support available to mothers within the community setting. A clinician's practice involves problem solving and interactions with mothers that may be related to an infant's latch, weight gain, or other areas of nutritional and health concerns.

In a support group setting, many mothers discuss how to overcome difficulties they encounter. In fact, support groups are often the places where mothers first go for support with difficulties and where problems might first be identified. This allows the intern to see how referrals come from mother-to-mother group leaders. Interns can not only observe mothers with breastfeeding problems, but also observe mothers who attend the group only for social support. This enables them to hear from mothers about developmental milestones, sleeping patterns, complementary feeding, and other typical events for babies as they grow. Exposure to normal, healthy children teaches an intern to learn to recognize situations that are not within normal limits.

ANTENATAL UNIT

Experience in an antenatal setting further develops an intern's teaching and counseling skills. A high-risk antenatal unit provides experience with expectant mothers who are likely to be receptive to learning about the health implications of providing their milk for their babies. The intern will also learn about the services and support systems available to these women. Every encounter with a mother is an extraordinary teachable moment, for both the mother and the intern.

BIRTH SETTINGS

Regardless of where the intern eventually practices, she will require an understanding of (and, if possible, exposure to) birthing environments. A mother's experiences during delivery and the early postpartum period can have a major impact on her decision to breast-feed and her long-term breastfeeding experience. When possible, internships should include exposure to births in a variety of

> **Consider...**
>
> Take advantage of every learning opportunity: One mother of trip-lets said that in her entire three-month-long hospital stay prior to the birth of her babies, no one came into her room to talk with her about breastfeeding.

healthcare settings (e.g., birth centers, community or referral hospitals), as well as home births and home visits during the early days or weeks of a child's life.

Observing intrapartum management and immediate postpartum care of the mother and child in a variety of birth settings provides insight into how a mother and her newborn subsequently experience breastfeeding. Immediately after birth, interns can participate in caring for the new mother by helping to place her baby skin to skin. She can point out the various stages a newborn experiences as he recovers from birth, adapts to the extrauterine world, and begins to breastfeed. If observation in these environments is not possible, special effort should be made to have the intern listen to mothers' descriptions of their birth experiences, how they perceived the care they received, and the mothers' own interpretation about the impact this may have had on her breastfeeding experience. There are also print and multimedia sources for exploring this progression.

Should the mother and her child need to be separated immediately after birth, it may provide an excellent opportunity for an intern to learn how to teach the mother to hand express her colostrum for the baby and why this could be helpful. If pumping is an option, the intern can help the mother begin to use the pump to trigger the onset of lactogenesis II.

> The clinical instructor can point out the importance of counseling skills and recognition of nonverbal communication to help the intern determine the mother's readiness for and response to teaching.

EARLY POSTPARTUM

Much of the intern's time should be spent helping mothers with breastfeeding during their first few days postpartum. Mothers' experiences and the quality of their breastfeeding during the first days postpartum may have an impact on meeting their long-term breastfeeding goals. The support and assistance a mother receives during this vulnerable time may influence her view of breastfeeding and whether she attains her breastfeeding goals. This time may determine her ability to establish full milk production and to learn effective breastfeeding management skills, and, therefore, provides the intern with many valuable lessons.

> **Consider...**
>
> As the intern observes the mother breastfeeding and offers suggestions, she assesses how well her suggestion or intervention is accepted. This may be through observing any signs of comfort or discomfort in the mother's body language and eye contact, or by asking the mother for feedback. She can also determine the mother's readiness for further help and teaching.

This environment enables interns to begin learning the process of taking a lactation history that includes pregnancy and birth, as well as previous medical and/or physical issues, medications, and surgeries the mother or child has encountered that could affect their breastfeeding. Taking repetitive histories from multiple mothers helps the intern recognize a variety of causes for a presenting problem, such as nipple soreness. A detailed history prepares the intern to individualize an appropriate plan of care for each mother and/or child. It instills an appreciation for data gathering, careful assessment, and analyzing information and insights.

Observing a mother's body language during history taking will signal the degree of comfort the mother has in answering personal questions. Perceived negative body language and avoidance of eye contact could have cultural roots, and an understanding of cultural nuances will help the intern determine this as the cause. It could also indicate a possible history of sexual, physical, or emotional abuse. If observed, the intern should continue with less sensitive history questions and defer to her clinical instructor.

> **Consider...**
>
> If a mother is uncomfortable learning to breast-feed with others present, the intern can invite visitors to leave and return after the feeding. They can be directed to a waiting room, with a promise to call them when the baby is done feeding. Some mothers may be uncomfortable making this request themselves for fear of offending a friend or family member. This simple intervention reinforces for the mother that the intern is an advocate for the mother and her child.

Observing feeding sessions provides opportunities for the intern to encounter a wide variety of feeding techniques and enhances her skills reading and interpreting nonverbal behavior. If the mother desires it, feeding sessions also provide a teachable opportunity to practice collaborative family-centered care by drawing other family members into the conversation, discussion, and suggested care plan. If the intern senses that a mother is uncomfortable, she may need to validate this perception, explore the source of the discomfort, and attempt to resolve it.

SPECIAL CARE NURSERY/NEONATAL INTENSIVE CARE

Exposure to the care of high-risk infants is an essential component of the intern's clinical experience. Working with infants and mothers in a special care nursery or a NICU setting offers insight into a mother's stress and its possible effect on her ability to express milk, to produce adequate amounts of milk, to normalize infant feeding, and to parent her child. Acquiring the skills learned helping a mother put a small, preterm infant to her breast will serve the intern in other aspects of her practice. Special care settings also provide opportunities to work with multidisciplinary healthcare teams assisting term babies who have an initial health challenge. In regions where milk banking is available, many special care nurseries use donor milk, as well as fortifiers and feeding modalities that the intern is not likely to see in any other clinical setting.

OTHER AREAS WITHIN A HOSPITAL

Breastfeeding mothers and children admitted to other areas within a hospital, such as pediatrics, medical, or surgical units, need to be recognized and supported. A health condition requiring admission has a tremendous potential for negative impact on breastfeeding in the absence of skilled assistance and support. The intern can gain valuable insights into working with very complicated situations often involving a team of healthcare providers. The healthcare team may involve representatives from the pharmacy, surgical and/or medical units, radiology, nutrition, social work, or infection control. Exposure to these multidisciplinary teams while the intern has skilled clinical instructors to guide and support her provides important experiences. Whenever the clinical instructor receives a referral to areas other than the maternity area, the intern should be included. The more unscheduled, unpredictable situations in which the intern participates, the better prepared and flexible she will be when practicing on her own.

OUTPATIENT LACTATION CLINIC

Most hospital-based IBCLCs spend the majority of their time caring for mothers and infants on the postpartum mother/baby unit and, for medical facilities with an outpatient clinic, consulting with breastfeeding dyads after discharge from the birth setting. The majority of the children seen in an outpatient visit are less than three months old. An instructor needs to be watchful for specific clinical situations involving older children to provide sufficient experiences for the intern. In a hospital setting providing only in-hospital based lactation services, it will be difficult to provide sufficient experiences with older children or with maternal conditions most frequently encountered beyond the immediate postpartum period. The intern will benefit from experiences with breastfeeding children of all ages.

PRIVATE PRACTICE

An IBCLC in private practice will experience a different type of clinic setting, and ideally home visits as well. Comparison of private clinical practice to that of an institutional setting helps the intern differentiate between the care provided in both settings and clinical situations encountered in the community. The intern will also learn the nuances and challenges of running a business and building a private practice. Private practice experience is a viable alternative for hospitals with no outpatient services.

PLANNING NONCLINICAL ACTIVITIES

Interns benefit from exposure to a variety of external business activities related to IBCLC clinical practice. Knowledge of ordering supplies, dealing with vendors, preparing a budget, creating monthly and yearly reports, and compliance with local and regional laws regulating practice all help the intern as she begins her own clinical practice. Other valuable experiences include attending meetings, learning to manage time, creating and maintaining client files, creating care plans and learning telephone time management.

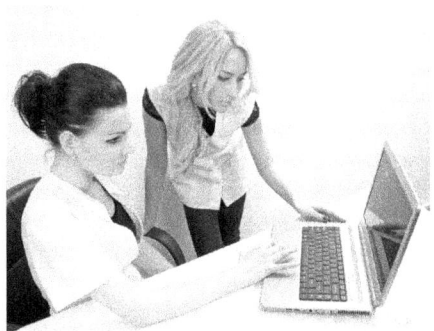

Figure 4.9 Interns need experience with a variety of nonclinical activities.

PROFESSIONAL MEETINGS

Inclusion of an intern in professional meetings with the clinical instructor will contribute to the intern's growth, especially within the workplace. The intern can gain invaluable insights observing interactions among various members of the healthcare team and hospital administration. Where available, encourage attendance at breastfeeding-related meetings for professionals. Breastfeeding advocacy occurs in many communities through multidisciplinary groups, such as coalitions that work collaboratively for health promotion. ILCA affiliates also meet in regions throughout the world. Encourage interns to attend meetings of mother-to-mother breastfeeding support groups, as well as similar support groups, such as those for mothers of multiples. Exposure to the larger community will broaden the intern's perspective as a practicing IBCLC. Such experience will help her be a more effective advocate for mothers and children effectively.

> **Consider...**
>
> The world of IBCLCs involves more than clinical care.

DOCUMENTATION

Accurate documentation in the mother's and child's health records throughout the internship is an important skill to be developed in the intern. Appendix 6 contains several samples of forms for documenting history, observations, and assessments. Orientation to the documentation method for each clinical site assures that the intern knows what is expected. Interns can begin by reading charts of previous patients with the instructor. The intern can analyze what is written and consider legalities and whether it will remain useful over a long period of time. This is especially relevant in the event that records become part of a court proceeding later in the child's life. The intern may not have considered legal aspects of documentation, and this will help her appreciate the need for accurate, complete, objective, and detailed documentation, including the use of standard abbreviations approved for use in her region of practice.

Teach interns to avoid charting meaningless statements, such as "discussed plan of care" or "made rounds." Documentation needs to describe specifically what was discussed or what was found during rounds. If the mother was asleep each time the intern attempted to visit, she can document, "mother was asleep" for each attempt. The use of correct, professional medical terminology is another important teaching point. Teach interns to avoid the use of nonprofessional colloquial jargon to describe signs and symptoms. They might quote exact words used by the mother. For example, they could document "bruising on the areola" or quote, "The mother states she has a hickie on the areola." It is imperative to note feedings observed with a description of the latch and the effectiveness of milk transfer during the feeding. Clear documentation also communicates the plan of care, expected timeframe for re-evaluation, and whether the IBCLC or mother will initiate the next evaluation step (e.g., "mother to phone in report" or "follow-up appointment scheduled for...").

Institutions that use electronic medical records will require the clinical instructor to supervise the intern's documentation. Documentation that includes narrative notes requires the clinical instructor to review the intern's narrative before it is posted. Interns tend to write everything that occurred during a consultation and will need guidance in learning to condense the narrative into concise descriptions. Narrative notes need to be consistent with other notations. For example, notes cannot reflect "good latch" in one entry and "shallow latch and difficulty staying on the breast" in another. Some hospitals adopt specific terms for documenting quality of a feed so that all lactation and nursing staff use the same terminology. The intern will then do the same. Some healthcare facilities require both instructor and intern signatures on documentation. Others may allow the lactation clinical internship program to define the required supervision of documentation until the intern has demonstrated mastery.

WRITTEN INSTRUCTIONS TO MOTHERS

Practice writing care plans will help interns select the most important elements necessary for lactation management to avoid overwhelming the mother with instruction and detail. It will also aid her communication with mothers and improve her ability to anticipate the outcome of a plan, while giving her skills in thinking about other eventualities. Written instructions should be stated simply, using commonly understood words and focusing on the most important aspects of the recommendations being made. The intern should review the written instructions carefully with mothers to verify that the instructions were accurately understood and seem reasonable. Before the mother leaves the hospital, the intern can ask, "Do you still think this plan will work for you at home or is there anything we should adjust now?"

FLEXIBILITY

Interns will learn they must put the mother's breastfeeding goals before their own. During her clinical placements, the intern will learn there is more than one way of viewing situations and that mothers will not always want to do what is recommended. The intern may have to accept a less than optimal plan of care or outcome that reflects a mother's abilities, needs, and desires. Additionally, mothers often present with more than one issue to be addressed. Being alert to all possible issues and learning to expect the unexpected will give the intern an appreciation that the career of an IBCLC is never boring!

TELEPHONE EXPERIENCES

Interns should answer lactation-related phone calls to respond to breastfeeding questions and make appointments. They can begin by listening while the clinical instructor communicates with mothers over the phone. They can then review the conversation and why it developed as it

> **Consider ...**
>
> One intern said "phone fear" was the scariest part of her internship. She worried she would say the wrong thing and the mother would hang up on her. This illustrates how interns react differently to experiences in their internship. No clinical instructor knows ahead of time what will be the most difficult for each of them.

did. Telephone triage is an important skill for the intern to develop. She will learn to identify circumstances when it is appropriate to give information and suggestions over the phone and which circumstances require an assessment and evaluation by the IBCLC or referral to another healthcare professional. Telephone conversations also present excellent opportunities to practice counseling skills. The intern can be guided to begin by asking open-ended questions and to focus the conversation with more probing and clarifying questions, while keeping the phone conversation to a reasonable time limit. This will become easier for the intern as she learns the art of phone triage.

SUMMARY

A good internship is much more than recording an intern's clinical hours. It provides opportunities for interns to practice in a variety of settings and across the entire skill set of IBCLC competencies. It is especially important that internships be focused on preparing participants for clinical problem solving. Regardless of the length of the internship, there will always be clinical situations not encountered that will present during some point in the IBCLC's professional practice. Both the internship and certification examination must assure that the candidate is able to safely address the required basics of lactation consulting and perform as a professional healthcare provider and team member.

Chapter 5

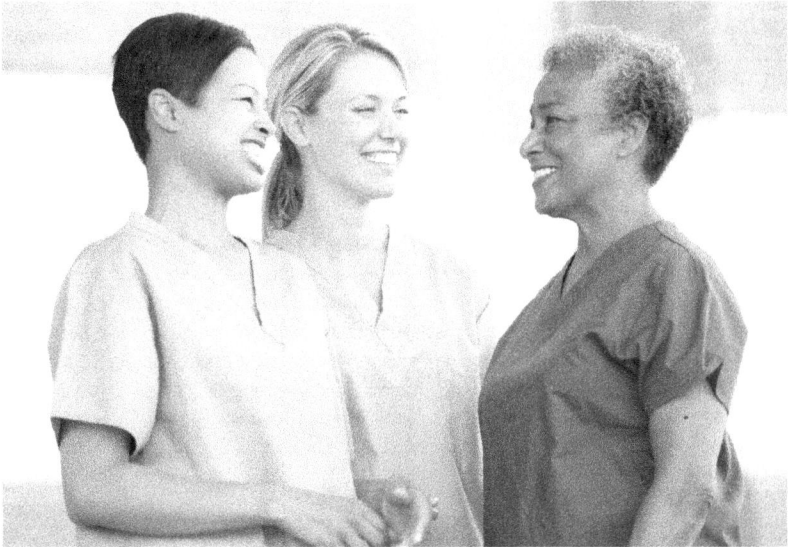

The Internship Experience

One of the most important elements of the intern-instructor relationship is the explicitly expressed and demonstrated confidence and belief in the intern. This confidence and willingness to make the commitment are demonstrated by spending the time and energy necessary (investing in the intern) to assure the intern's success. Much can be learned from the thoughtful feedback of interns. In retrospect, they are able to identify strengths that they brought to the internship, challenges they faced, and areas within the internship that may need modification. Most of the information in this text evolved over many experiences with the input of interns, colleagues, and multidisciplinary teammates. These recommendations are tried and true, but, of course, not necessarily the only way to do things.

The instructor's willingness to spend time and energy, and to commit to demonstrating confidence in the capabilities of the intern to think critically, is important in both informal interactions and formal evaluations. The instructor should prepare the intern to be challenged to explain her rationale, and then to consider and defend alternative actions. There is no one right way to do most of lactation consulting. What is right today may later be disputed when new research points to another more effective approach. Teaching interns critical thinking processes rather than facts and rules permits interns access to the growth opportunities within the future of this young profession. Awareness of alternatives, intentional thought processes, and decision making are all part of the critical thinking process that instructors hope to instill in those who come to them for clinical instruction.

> **Intern Grad Tip**
>
> "After completing the first 200 hours of my part-time internship, I felt I had a brief exposure to the true world of lactation support. I not only wanted more experience and clinical hours, but I knew I needed this precious on-site time to grow and prepare myself for these skills in the field. I decided to enter … a full-time internship course … This decision was ultimately made because of the growing faith and confidence my mentors had in me. The timely feedback through weekly evaluations, one-on-one meetings, and discussions with my mentors are how I have been able to measure my own progress as an intern. I am able to understand my strengths and weaknesses and build focus for improvement every day."

STARTING THE INTERNSHIP

How an internship starts will vary somewhat by the setting. There are common elements that occur in each. Before any clinical instruction takes place, the intern needs to receive an orientation to the clinical sites and to the expectations of the internship. This will include the elements of standard employee orientation to the facility, introductions to other staff, explanations of the intern's role, and agreement on the intern's schedule. Throughout the internship, scheduling, planning for different experiences, reviewing progress, and evaluations will be subject to change as the intern's needs evolve. However, an initial orientation will set the ground rules and provide a clear definition of expectations.

INTERN ORIENTATION

The internship should begin with an intern orientation. An orientation program may be similar to the way other healthcare students are oriented to a facility or practice. It is essential to provide a written participant handbook of applicable institutional policies (see Appendix 3). It is recommended the intern provide written acknowledgement of receiving the handbook and receive a certificate of completion of the orientation. The intern should also receive a course syllabus with explanations about the experiences needed to progress. She will begin with observation, and then progress to more independent practice when she is ready. Readiness to progress to direct care occurs more quickly with basic skills than with more complex skills or clinical situations. Elements of an intern orientation are described in Figure 5.1.

Figure 5.1 Elements of the Intern Orientation

- Brief tour of exit locations.
- Safety, emergency, and security procedures.
- Within hospital settings, use of a badge identifying the intern's role provides access to protected locations, such as labor and delivery, the mother-baby unit/ward, and special care nurseries.
- How to contact the instructor(s) or colleagues, from both within and outside the facility.
- Computer and phone access and instruction, including logins, e-mail access, and access to any shared file systems and electronic medical record keeping system.
- Written work to be submitted, when it is expected, and how much is required.
- The intern's responsibility for keeping accurate, up-to-date time logs, and what to expect of the evaluation process (who will do it, how often, etc.).
- What to do in case of illness or emergency.
- How disciplinary actions are handled.
- The dress code, rules for appearance applicable to the units where the intern may be working (e.g., jewelry, perfume, artificial nails, hair), common misconceptions, and unit-based exceptions.

SCHEDULING

Scheduling is accomplished collaboratively with all the participating instructors. Written copies of the schedule are posted or provided to each instructor, as well as the intern. Depending on the availability of the instructors, certain days and times may be difficult to schedule when the amount of teaching requires a slower pace. When they are scheduled in the clinical area two days each week, many interns anticipate they will have free time the rest of the week for family responsibilities, other educational endeavors, or employment. Due to the amount of required written work, the potential for outside research or study, and other learning activities, this expectation may be unrealistic. Reviewing these requirements during orientation will prepare the interns for the amount of work to anticipate.

> **Intern Grad Tip**
>
> "In preparing for a lactation consultant internship, consider it similar to a full-time job. For every hour you spend with patients, expect to spend at least two hours in charting, didactics, research, and discussions with your clinical instructors. Take your time; this is not a portion of your education which you want to rush."

In a practice setting where several instructors share the responsibility for teaching, scheduling one or more interns with the instructor every day can lead to burnout, regardless of the instructor's workload and other responsibilities. Fast paced, busy practices will need to make adjustments in staffing patterns to accommodate teaching of lactation consultant interns early in their internship. Further along, interns are able to participate in more care with less intensive supervision. The presence of advanced interns allows for larger numbers of mothers and children to be seen in less time, freeing the instructor for other responsibilities. Near the end of an internship, it is essential the instructor be available for onsite supervision to allow for immediate collaboration with the intern. Such collaboration helps the intern learn measures and management skills to promptly and professionally handle unexpected events or situations that suddenly become more complex, or in which unexpected complications or issues arise.

INTRODUCTIONS AND EXPLAINING THE INTERN'S ROLE

At every opportunity, the intern should be introduced to the multidisciplinary team. It is helpful to include information detailing when the intern will be present and what her current role entails. The instructor can explain her role to the rest of the staff as that of guiding, teaching, and providing feedback to the intern. Introductions to each client/family should be made as a matter of courtesy, including the role of the intern and that she is preparing for IBCLC certification.

In settings that require a signed consent for treatment (e.g., outpatient clinic visits), it is appropriate to point out that this is consent for treatment by both the instructor and intern. If a particular family objects to having an intern involved in their care, the instructor can speak with them first to explain the intern's and instructor's roles. If the family still objects, the intern can be assigned to other duties.

IN THE BEGINNING: FIRST EXPERIENCES

The intern will begin her clinical experience by observing the clinical instructor as the instructor provides care to mothers and babies. This initial phase of observation is critical to the intern's self-confidence and professional growth. As the intern's confidence increases, and when the instructor considers the intern ready to progress beyond observation, the intern will begin direct supervised contact with mothers and babies. When ready, the intern will then proceed to working independently, with the instructor available to assist as needed.

BRIEFINGS AND DEBRIEFINGS

Brief meetings between the instructor and intern at the beginning and end of the clinical day help structure the intern's learning. These may be frequent early in the internship and can decrease as the intern progresses. At the beginning of the clinical day, the instructor and intern can sit down to briefly review what to anticipate for the day. This will give the intern time to research a particular clinical topic prior to seeing a dyad with an unfamiliar condition. It also gives the opportunity for questions and clarifying any issues before beginning the day. Debriefing at the end of the clinical day may include a review of any encounters that raised questions or issues for the intern.

PROGRESSION FROM OBSERVATION TO INDEPENDENT PRACTICE

There are two descriptions of the progressive paths that interns follow as they move from simply observing to performing a complete consultation alone. These descriptions help the clinical instructor understand how participation, practice, and development of self-confidence are necessary as the intern progresses from one level to the next.

Table 5.1 shows the three phases of participation as described by IBLCE and adapted by the authors (IBLCE, 2011c). This progression will be individualized according to particular clinical situations. For example, the intern may be ready to progress more quickly to helping mothers with latch or hand expression, but may need more time in earlier stages with more complicated clinical situations.

Table 5.1. Three Phases of Intern Participation in Directly Supervised Clinical Practice

PHASE ONE	• The intern's role is restricted to observation of the supervising IBCLC and taking notes for her own use. • The clinical instructor needs to allot time after a consultation to debrief and ask the intern what she learned and if she has any questions. • This is a good time to ask the intern to explain the rationale for what the IBCLC said and did as an exercise in using and developing her critical thinking skills.
PHASE TWO	• The intern works directly with breastfeeding families under the direct supervision of the supervising IBCLC. • The intern takes the history, completes written forms, and does a physical assessment of both the mothers and infants. • The clinical instructor does the feeding assessment and develops the plan of care. • This phase progresses into the intern doing the complete consult with the clinical instructor watching.
PHASE THREE	• The intern practices independently, with the supervising IBCLC on site and available to assist if needed. • The intern does the entire consult with the clinical instructor out of the room. • At the end of the consult, the intern succinctly presents her findings, including the plan of care to her instructor. • The instructor approves the assessment and plan of care and includes her signature along with the intern's signature on the assessment form. This allows the mother or insurance company to be billed for the consult. • The intern does all the follow-up paperwork.

Source: IBLCE, 2011c.

Table 5.2 describes four stages that the intern will move through as she learns to be a lactation consultant: Anticipatory, Formal, Informal, and Personal. Interns will progress through the four stages of role acquisition in varying lengths of time. They cannot be pushed faster than they are able to move. Instructors can model personal stage behavior to help them grasp the need for flexibility in developing their plan of care for mothers and babies. The information is adapted from a model of parental role acquisition written by Debi Bocar and Karen Moore (Barger, 2002).

Table 5.2. Acquiring the Lactation Consultant Role

ANTICIPATORY STAGE	• The aspiring lactation consultant collects information from many different sources. She may have come in contact with other lactation consultants during her own breastfeeding career or may have read about IBCLCs in a book or magazine. She may want to do something "different" that she can do with young children. She may love breastfeeding and want to work with breastfeeding mothers. She may have worked with experienced lactation consultants in a hospital setting, with breastfeeding women in a public health clinic, or with a mother-to-mother support group, and now wants to formalize her training and experience. • She makes the decision to pursue this goal and begins to collect information on how to do it through talking to others; contacting ILCA, IBLCE, and course providers; resources in books or magazines; and other sources of information. • She probably has a fairly idealized picture of herself as a lactation consultant, working out of her home with plenty of time for her family, making plenty of money, or finding a perfect job in a clinic or hospital. • She completes a lactation management program in preparation for obtaining clinical experience.
FORMAL STAGE	• The intern enters a lactation consultant internship and begins to assume responsibility for caring for mothers and infants. This may seem intimidating to those who have not had direct contact with mothers and infants in a professional setting. A nurse or other healthcare provider who has been caring for women routinely may need to change her thinking and the way she approaches breastfeeding. • The intern relies on formalized expectations of a lactation consultant as stated in objective, written terms in a job description, standards of practice (ILCA, 2006), and professional ethics (IBLCE, 2011b). • The intern begins to break down preconceived ideas and teaching, and may teach colleagues what she has learned and believes they need to know.

FORMAL STAGE CONTINUED	• The intern finds there is conflicting advice among the "experts." She wants to do everything the "right" and "best" way, and is nonplussed to discover that there may be as many "right" and "best" ways as there are experts. She finds it frustrating to have learned one method of doing things in her lactation management class, only to learn yet another way in her internship. Having to choose from more than one method may feel overwhelming to her • Lactation management may be rigidly and formally performed, trying to do it "right." She will be sensitive to comments and nonverbal cues from those she perceives as "experts." • Though the intern is eager to do things on her own, she feels safer watching others do it or having someone nearby. She may feel inadequate, demonstrate low self-confidence, and require reassurance that each task she undertakes was done correctly. It is important to give the intern a great deal of moral support and affirmation that she has done the best for that mother and child • This is a difficult time for making decisions based on the individual mother and child's needs, as the intern may view problem analysis and planning care in black and white. For example, when helping a mother with engorgement, she will have to sort through conflicting recommendations regarding the use of cabbage. She will have learned that applying cabbage leaves over a prolonged period of time can dry up the mother's milk. She has read in a professional journal that cabbage applied for 20 minutes three to four times a day to treat engorgement did not work. It would be hard for the intern at this stage to extrapolate that using cabbage until the mother experiences relief from the engorgement is acceptable practice. • By the end of this stage, the intern trusts that she is adequately performing the essential plans of care and feels comfortable with new mothers. She no longer believes she must know everything and is confident with more than one approach to situations. For some this occurs during a clinical internship; for others it may not occur until the individual is practicing independently.
INFORMAL STAGE	• The intern begins to modify the rigid rules and directions she sought out and used during the formal stage. She begins to put together the different approaches to care she has learned and is willing to consider other options. • This is a great stage for the intern to begin to interact in a forum. She can learn ways to approach clinical situations in an online forum such as Lactnet (2012) or the ILCA blog, Lactation Matters (2012b). • The intern's interactions with mothers and other lactation consultants may become more spontaneous, with less fear of imperfection.

PERSONAL STAGE	• The intern further evolves her role to a style consistent with her own personality. • The intern is better able to handle individuality among new mothers and is not as quick to assume that if the mother stops breastfeeding it is her fault. She is more comfortable with a mother who chooses an alternative path that the lactation consultant may not consider "optimal." • The intern is more willing to consider other options and seek out others' opinions, quickly discarding them if they are incompatible with her personal approach. • The intern is able to read and critique research, accepting what she considers applicable and discarding what is not. • The intern is comfortable in her role and relishes the opportunity to teach others. • This stage often is not reached during a clinical internship.

Source: Barger, 2002.

OBSERVATIONAL EXPERIENCES

As the intern begins the observation phase of the internship, it is critical to instruct the intern when it is and is not acceptable to talk during the interaction. This can be challenging for talkative or enthusiastic individuals. It may be helpful to establish a code word or subtle gesture ahead of time that serves as a reminder when to remain quiet.

Use of a model for feeding observation (for example, see Breastfeeding Observation Form in Appendix 6) will help interns focus their feeding observations. During initial observations, the instructor may want to identify what to anticipate and what the priorities are during the client interaction just before entering the client's presence. The intern can be asked to take notes, for example, and to watch the mother's body language and how she holds her child.

Figure 5.2 presents a model of brief questions to ask the intern immediately after an observation to help her process what she observed. A model that has brief post-interaction questions provides a consistent way to focus observation experiences. This process has been most helpful early in the program to help the intern understand what has happened and what it meant. The instructor may point out specific ways the interaction was individualized, or what directed her to select one approach over another.

Figure 5.2. Exit Questions for Observations

1. How do you feel the visit/interaction went overall?
2. What is one thing that was positive or effective about the visit?
3. What is one thing that might have been more effective if done differently?
4. What is the next step?

PROGRESSING FROM OBSERVATION TO INCREASED PARTICIPATION

The amount of time spent in observation before progressing to direct care will vary with each intern and with individual clinical situations. The intern should be able to explain the rationale for the care she observed given by the instructor. She should also routinely identify major observations and relevant elements for the history, assessment, and plan of care. As interns reach this threshold, they are ready to begin participating in caring for mothers and babies. Some interns may need assistance gaining confidence to move from observation to direct care. Briefings before and debriefings immediately after clinical encounters will help the intern synthesize what occurs and provide an opportunity for brief questions to help direct the intern's learning.

As direct care begins, the instructor and intern may share components of each interaction. For example, the intern might record the history and assessment as they are performed by the instructor. After she masters this, she may be given responsibility for writing the plan of care as the instructor dictates it. She can then write any necessary follow-up reports. When this level of participation has been mastered, the intern can then begin doing the history, assessment, and plan of care while the instructor observes. This stage usually requires additional time, which needs to be factored into the intern's schedule (perhaps 30 minutes for each encounter). When this level of participation is mastered, the intern can move to working independently, with the instructor available as needed.

There is a wide variety of personalities among lactation interns and instructors, as with any group of people. Self-awareness and being suitably qualified will help the instructor meet the learning needs of each intern. Tools, such as written scripts, note cards, and index-card-sized standard care plans, can be kept in a pocket for quick reference to help the intern who is beginning to practice providing care on her own. If an intern is hesitant to participate in a particular skill, the instructor might find role-playing helpful, with the instructor playing the part of the mother.

INTERN PREFERENCE

At times an intern will want to begin by first going into the mother's room by herself. The instructor can enter later to review what she has done and provide her "expert" agreement for the mother's benefit. At other times, the intern may prefer that the instructor begin the interaction with her. The instructor can then ease out as the intern is comfortable continuing to observe the remainder of a feeding on her own and establish a plan for follow up. Most of this will need to be individualized and may need adjustment, dictated by both the intern's and the mother's comfort level.

CLINICAL SETTING

The intern's direct involvement will vary depending on the clinical setting. In the NICU, the instructor may never be more than a few feet away, whereas in

s Clinical Instruction in Lactation

a mother-baby unit she may be at the nurses' desk or in another room. During outpatient visits, the instructor may start out in a room nearby for easy access.

CASE REVIEW

Later in the internship, the instructor may appear at a prearranged time to review the case and care options with the intern and mother. In most cases, it is appropriate to conduct this review in the presence of the mother (and family) as a way to summarize, reinforce, and make sure that in providing instruction to the mother, both teaching and learning occurred.

Just as with any form of communication, what is said is not always the same as what is heard. A care provider may believe she taught a concept, but because of a wide variety of influences on communication, learning may not have occurred. Many healthcare environments use models that recommend limiting teaching to three primary points at a time. This increases the likelihood that the learner will more easily remember and retain the information. The learner can also be asked to restate what was taught in her own words, as though she were explaining to another family member (this is the "teach-back" model).

WRITTEN ASSIGNMENTS

Written work should be an essential element incorporated into lactation clinical internships to provide validation of the intern's knowledge and understanding (Figure 5.3). Activities include written exercises that reflect understanding of didactic learning and its application to clinical conditions. Later, written work throughout the internship provides opportunities to record and analyze the quality of clinical interactions. These activities are crucial to the intern's growth and instructors are urged to incorporate them into their lactation internships.

VALIDATION OF DIDACTIC KNOWLEDGE

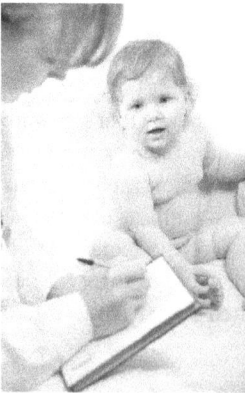

Figure 5.3. Written assignments help validate the intern's understanding.

The first purpose of written work in a lactation clinical internship is to validate the intern's knowledge and her understanding of how to apply what she learned in the lactation specific course-work she has completed. This is an important part of the preparation the intern must complete prior to observations in the clinical setting. For example, the workbook, *Clinical Experiences in Lactation: A Blueprint for Internship, 3rd edition* (Kutner & Barger, 2010), contains a section about various maternal and infant conditions that may impact lactation. The first page for each condition is a "didactic" or summary worksheet about that condition, its causes, and possible approaches to lactation management. See Appendix 4 for samples of these worksheets for hyperbilirubinemia and engorgement.

Analyzing typical causes and treatments for commonly experienced clinical problems prompts the intern to synthesize what she has been exposed to in her own reading, background experiences, and lactation coursework. An intern may find herself overwhelmed by information from different sources. What appears to be conflicting advice may simply represent options for different approaches. This is where the use of index card (3"x5") standard care plans will help the intern distill all the hours of study into "top three priorities" for different conditions.

The instructor will need to guide the intern as to an appropriate length for written work. She should specify the resources and references that are acceptable and clarify how references are to be cited. Programs with large numbers of interns will need to balance the amount of written work required with the instructor(s) available dedicated time for reviewing the written work and discussing it with the interns.

ANALYSIS OF CLINICAL EXPERIENCES

Interns can use written analysis of experiences and case reports to record impressions during observations, and later to record and analyze their clinical interactions with mothers and babies. Such analysis provides the opportunity for the intern to reflect on clinical practice as she evaluates interventions and enhances her problem-solving skills. The frequency with which interns record experiences can be negotiated between the intern and instructor. It is probably not necessary that an intern write up every client interaction. Perhaps recording a couple of client experiences at the end

> **Intern Grad Tip**
>
> "As you finish your didactic learning, have some sort of portable reference (pocket notebook, flashcards, electronic device) where you can summarize main ideas and list defining/distinguishing characteristics or typical symptoms to use as a quick resource when you are faced with a new scenario."

of each clinical day will provide the necessary analysis to represent seminal or unique learning experiences during that day. Over the course of the internship, the intern and clinical instructor need to have a record keeping system, so they can review what types of experiences the intern should be having, analyzing, and writing.

To fully utilize the limited number of hours the intern is with the instructor, it is important to maximize the learning that occurs during that time. Written work requires dedicated time to review, comment, and then discuss this work with the intern. To be most effective, written work needs to be done relatively concurrent with the experience. Neither the instructor nor the intern will recall details and nuances if too much time has elapsed. It is also important that the instructor who was present for the client interaction be the one to review the written work related to that experience, making the most of the instructor's familiarity with details of the case and the experience. Figure 5.4 describes other possible written activities.

Figure 5.4. Other Written Activities

- Describe clinical events you observed today. Reflect on those where you learned something unexpected and your accompanying thoughts and feelings. What concepts can you generalize for future application?

- Describe the most significant event that occurred today. Indicate what you learned from the experience, how you would behave the next time in a similar situation, and how your didactic learning provides guidance for action (Burrows, 1995).

- Identify learning goals in advance and evaluate them at the end of the day. Analyze the day's events and critically connect theory to practice. Reflect on your clinical experiences and your attitudes and feelings associated with them (Ruthman, 2004).

- Reflect on your newborn assessment and compare it to what you anticipated. What significant differences did you find? What implications can you derive for future assessments (Ruthman, 2004)?

MANAGING WRITTEN WORK

While there may be clinical internships that do not incorporate written work, it is not advisable. The shared client experience as described on paper by the lactation consultant intern may bring to the instructor's attention important elements that have been missed or misinterpreted. This is also a consideration to be addressed when setting up situations for clinical instructors to supervise internship experiences at a distance. Even with the use of video, voice over internet protocols (e.g., Skype, etc.), or other electronic media, the instructor will not have the same sensory input as the intern who is on site. Transmitting data and electronic media must be by secure networks to protect the privacy of the mothers and children and meet government regulations.

In development of the internship program, decisions need to be made about how and when these written elements are to be presented and processed (e.g., handwritten, electronic, etc.). A record keeping system needs to be established for tracking the assignments. While these are primarily the responsibility of the intern, structural supports, such as the use of checklists and forms, can help the intern keep appropriate and organized records that become part of the officially stored and retrievable academic records. This is especially important for interns working through an internship under IBLCE Pathway 3 program, where the verification of skill competencies and hours in supervised practice is an essential element for the completion of that pathway.

TOPICS TO DISCUSS DURING INTERNSHIPS

During the course of a lactation internship, specific topics need to be addressed which may or may not have been part of the intern's didactic learning prior to the clinical component. These include essential information and examples of application of the theoretical information to which they may have already been exposed. Appendix 1 includes sample topics to review with interns during such educational conferences, including ethics, healthcare privacy, burnout, and dealing with challenging communication situations. While these need not be complex, they do need to be explained clearly to the intern. Throughout the internship, it is helpful if the instructor points out specific examples of how these topics apply and relates them to the clinical practice of lactation consulting.

TEACHING COUNSELING SKILLS

Teaching interns how to manage clinical situations and find solutions to breastfeeding challenges is the easy part of the internship. More challenging is helping the intern to refine her communication skills and to use counseling techniques effectively with mothers. Attention to counseling skills can be difficult, especially for healthcare professionals who may be quick to fix a problem and less accustomed to sitting and listening. In the beginning, the intern may not be aware of the instructor's use of counseling skills, and may see it as social conversation or pleasantries. This illustrates why the postconsult debriefing with the intern is so important. It allows the instructor and the intern to discuss all the nuances of the interactions with mothers. They can review what was said and why, the mothers' responses and the possible reasons for those responses, and how the approach added to or detracted from the interaction. Developing effective counseling skills requires a lot of practice, and the progress toward acquisition of these skills should be a standard part of every evaluation conference.

Most clinical instructors will have to think about how to teach these skills, which may seem automatic to those who have been in practice for a period of time. It is helpful to think about how these skills are demonstrated and point that out to the intern in the clinical situation. Listening skills are not necessarily obvious to an observer, and probably need to be explicitly addressed. The importance of listening to what is and what is *not* said by a mother (or family), and the emotional content of what is said, need special attentiveness. The intern may need to be advised and guided to focus on attending to what is being communicated, rather than formulating what she wants to say next while the mother is talking.

Establishing relationships takes time and attention. These counseling skills will be essential for the intern, both in her interactions with mothers and families, as well as with professional colleagues. Asking questions during history taking, the use of open-ended questions, and the acknowledgement of emotional messages are all skills the intern needs to be aware of and receive explicit guidance about from the clinical instructor. The use of simulation, role play, and video recordings can be especially helpful in learning and evaluating these skills. An intern's previous background as a healthcare provider will not preclude this being an area to explore during a lactation internship, including the nuances specific to lactation clinical care. Many experienced practicing healthcare providers continue to work actively to refine communication and counseling skills with different populations, settings, and roles throughout their professional careers.

LANGUAGE AND TERMINOLOGY

The appropriateness of using the mothers' own language can be another element related to counseling skills. Using the mother's own words to describe body parts or situations can be an effective way to demonstrate acceptance and facilitate understanding. Sometimes this will not be comfortable or appropriate, and interns will need to find what works best for them. Interpretation services are important when the instructor's or the intern's language is not the mother's first language. It is recognized in general healthcare that use of family members for interpretation can be ineffective, and does not meet legal criteria of assuring informed care or professional communication.

Some medical interpreters may not be very familiar with breastfeeding, so it is important to make sure the meaning is clear by using examples and asking the mother and family to "teach back" what was discussed. In addition, it takes some skill and practice to become comfortable with using interpretation services effectively, making sure to use appropriate eye contact and touch, and to talk to the mother directly (not to the interpreter), using short, simple, direct communication.

LITERACY

Concepts related to healthcare terminology are also relevant. Many words and concepts used in the healthcare environment are not easily understood by the general public. Interns will benefit from practice at both oral and written client teaching which assesses effectiveness of learning by the mother and family. Teach practical approaches to making written instructions readable and useful for families with low literacy skills or low healthcare literacy. Limiting the amount of text on a page, simplifying essentials into no more than three major points, and asking the mother/family to explain back what they understood are useful techniques.

TEACHING ABOUT THE USE OF TOUCH

In cultures where it is embraced, the use of touch is a great adjunct to verbal interaction and can be used to convey caring. It is also an indispensable skill for physical examination of both mother and child. Touching without permission is a legal issue, and it is important that lactation interns be taught how legal consent for treatment and permission to touch is sought, as well as how necessary

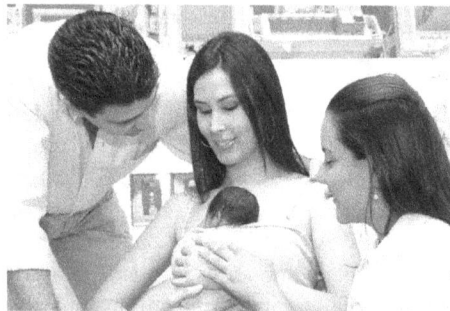

Figure 5.5. Instructors can help interns become comfortable with appropriate touch.

touch is explained and justified. Lactation interns need to develop the skill of appropriate touch that is individualized to specific circumstances and settings

(Figure 5.5). Some interns will need more time and practice to develop comfort using these skills than others. Interns with a healthcare background may be more comfortable with the use of touch, and for some this could result in using it more than is necessary. They may need help to understand how their touch is perceived and whether it might seem invasive.

Touching invades the mother's and child's personal space, so awareness of mothers' responses is essential. Teach interns to be alert to both verbal and nonverbal cues that may signal a need for the intern to adjust her approach. The prevalence of women with a history of being inappropriately touched (Simkin & Klaus, 2004) means that not all well-intentioned touch will be received positively.

TEACHING PHYSICAL EXAMINATION SKILLS

There is an enormous amount of information that can be obtained and elicited by observation and history taking. However, there is no substitute for a hands-on physical examination related to what is going on with both mothers and babies. The appropriate clinical skills for physical examinations should be demonstrated by the clinical instructor, with return demonstration by the intern. Clinical instructors who are skilled at physical assessment will need to think about the individual discreet steps they take in making assessments and observation, and rationale for those steps in performing physical assessments as part of lactation care.

Refining observational and hands-on skills requires time, exposure through demonstration, progressive guided practice, and opportunities to do it repeatedly. Clinical instructors will need to make opportunities for their own examinations to be repeated by the intern without being overwhelming to the mother and/or baby. Skilled instructors can use this as an opportunity to explain to the intern, as well as to the mother and her family, why certain things are done and what findings may indicate.

TEACHING ANALYSIS AND CRITICAL THINKING

Interns need to learn to think both intuitively and analytically. Regardless of the intern's learning style or the instructors' understanding of learning theories (e.g., right brain-left brain, etc.), lactation consultants are required to have the same clinical reasoning and problem-solving skills common to all healthcare providers. Effective teaching methods in the clinical area for advanced practice nurses (Truscott, 2010) and for doctors (Kassirer, 2010) share a common focus on the use of real-life clinical cases. A similar approach is useful for the preparation of lactation consultants.

The accuracy of problem identification and analysis, or diagnosis, is necessarily a prerequisite to understanding causes and possible solutions for problems. This type of analytical skill is used in many professions and most familiarly in healthcare to determine medical diagnoses. It is an essential skill to be taught during lactation internships. Accurate diagnosis (analysis of findings, recognition of problems) and an understanding of pathophysiology and causality increase the likelihood of selecting appropriate and effective treatments or strategies to resolve problems. Lactation interns and lactation consultants who develop this skill are less likely to make a standard recommendation to all mothers with similar presenting complaints.

Various types of treatment options and modalities are available to lactation consultants based on individual clinical situations. For example, sore nipples may have many different causes, and the treatment recommended would not be the same for all mothers. The lactation intern will need help from the clinical instructor to recognize the different causes and when the treatment for one mother might be ineffective or even harmful for another mother. It is critical to teach selection of treatment options in collaboration with the families receiving lactation care. The clinical instructor can coach the intern in how to determine acceptability of a plan of care to the mother and her family, with consideration of cost and feasibility of different recommendations, as well as meeting all the aspects of informed consent.

> **Consider...**
>
>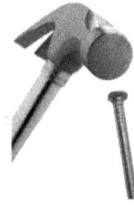
>
> If the only tool you have is a hammer, every problem looks like a nail.

> **Consider...**
>
> A mother with low milk production for her one-month-old baby has two preschool children or school-age children with after-school activities. A new lactation intern may have unrealistic expectations of the mother that fail to recognize the impact of her other children on her available time and energy. An experienced clinical instructor could suggest the intern list the various ways the mother might increase milk production, and work with the mother and her family on a collaborative plan that the *mother* considers reasonable

In the process of developing a care plan in conjunction with the mother, the intern will be guided through the process of helping the mother recognize positive outcomes. She will learn to anticipate the expected speed of resolving a problem, as well as when a return visit for follow-up would be appropriate. Again, the collaborative aspects of clinical caregiving must be emphasized. There is never one particular solution to a problem that will work for all mothers. When problems are misidentified or incompletely analyzed, the treatments recommended do not resolve the problem. The consequence of an inaccurate lactation diagnosis is inappropriate treatment, which will inevitably result in nonresolution of the problem. This could be one of the reasons mothers who have had a previous breastfeeding "failure" wish not to try again with subsequent children.

Analytical processes can be broken down into discrete steps: hypothesis, pattern recognition, interpretation of findings, differential diagnosis, and verification of diagnosis. The process is further described in Figure 5.6. Developing the intuitive part of this process leads to first impressions and pattern recognition becoming immediate, automatic, and almost instinctive. These skills are very difficult to teach in a classroom or lecture setting. However, the accumulation of unanalyzed clinical experiences also misses the mark of learning this skill, as a clinician can repeatedly make errors that go unrecognized if the process is not analyzed.

Case-based analysis with an experienced "coach" (clinical instructor) can be an expensive and time consuming process. Yet it remains a strongly recommended way to achieve purposeful learning (Kassirer, 2010). This illustrates why the simple accumulation of hours or clinical experiences is not an accurate measure of learning. *True learning is what occurs in the mind of the intern.* It is the job of the creative clinical instructor to provide the opportunities for learning, promoting, guiding, and assessing this learning process. This is done most effectively in real-life clinical practice situations, such as those encountered through an internship. For some rare conditions, simulations, recordings, role play, or case studies may be used as adjunct teaching methods.

Figure 5.6. The Process of Critical Thinking

- Applies reason and logic to ideas, opinions, and situations.
- Uses predictable logic that has a clear purpose.
- Questions assumptions and considers multiple perspectives.
- Analyzes information to support conclusions.
- Changes conclusions based on convincing evidence.
- Uses evidence to guide decisions.

EVALUATION

Ongoing feedback from instructors and interns is an essential component of the internship. Such evaluation helps identify the need to revise teaching strategies and techniques, revisit goals, and adjust the specific time frames and internship schedules as specific skills are mastered. To be most effective, this evaluation process should be bidirectional, with the intern also offering periodic feedback based on her self-assessment of skill development and the teaching strategies, modalities, and pace that work best for her. Examples of evaluation forms are provided in Appendix 5.

Evaluation is not necessarily a comfortable process for the intern, as the process of being challenged, questioned, and continually put into novel situations may challenge her coping skills. Individualization, as well as a respectful, nonthreatening environment, works best when the instructor is willing to process information along with the intern, acknowledging both the rewards and challenges inherent in clinical care giving. Pointing out an error in thinking or judgment in a respectful manner immediately after it occurs can be a great learning opportunity.

ROUTINE EVALUATIONS

In the beginning of the internship, it is recommended that written evaluations be conducted daily to identify clinical experiences encountered and evaluate the intern's mastery of skills. Frequency of these written evaluations can decrease as the intern progresses, first changing to weekly evaluations, then perhaps even to monthly, depending on the length and pace of the internship. The instructor's assessments should focus on the intern's strengths, as well as areas needing improvement. The instructor can also point out progress the intern has made since the previous evaluation.

EVALUATING OUTCOMES

Determining outcomes of the internship should be an explicit part of the design of the program. Written work and other records kept by both the intern and the clinical instructor help to establish documentation of the intern's competence. The *Clinical Competencies Checklist* in Appendix 4 or a similar checklist can be used for this purpose. Records should note when alternative strategies were used to review topics or experiences that were unavailable during the clinical internship. Some of these may have been made available at other sites, and the evaluation of the effectiveness of those experiences and processes must also be undertaken on a regular basis.

EVALUATING OFFSITE INSTRUCTORS

Often lactation consultant internship programs are designed using offsite clinical instructors who are IBCLCs in practice in nearby or remote communities. In these cases, the coordinator of the program will also evaluate those instructors' teaching abilities, as well as the strengths and challenges unique to their specific clinical site. Accountability and the types of support, communications, compensation, and other services offered to instructors are a consideration during the program design.

FINAL EVALUATIONS

The final evaluation process at the end of an internship should be bidirectional, with the instructor(s) offering comments about the intern's strengths, as well as recommendations for further preparation that might be necessary before pursuing certification, and any for future growth and learning. The intern should have an opportunity to give both formal and informal evaluation of each instructor, as well as the overall program, and to complete a final self-evaluation of skill competence/mastery at the closure of the internship.

PROGRAM COMPLETION

The internship program should issue the graduating intern a designated statement, letter, or certificate of completion. Educational records charting the progress of internship hours and skills, copies of all evaluations, and other intern materials should be filed for retrieval and verification as needed. When internships are not part of an educational institution, the program design will need to address secure storage of educational records and processes to facilitate retrieval of records.

SUMMARY

The internship experience is defined by how well designed the program is. The pace and depth of experiences vary dramatically from one setting to another. A well-designed and organized program maximizes learning opportunities and provides for progressive skill development through the process of ongoing analysis and evaluation. The future of the lactation consulting profession requires attention to development and standardization of high quality clinical instruction and best practices.

Chapter 6

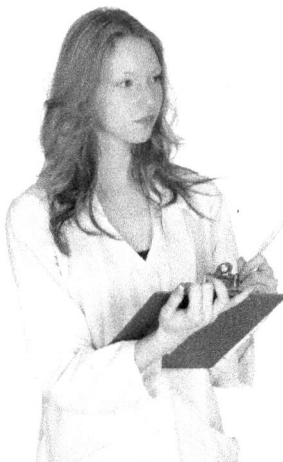

Internship Models

Educators who provide lactation management courses are in a prime position to offer information about clinical internship options. Some programs provide their own internships. Referrals to internships often come by word of mouth from one professional to another and from one student or intern to another. ILCA and other professional groups, such as breastfeeding coalitions, can also be an effective means for referral of potential clinical internship candidates. Networking through social media, electronic information and databases, and informal channels, such as blogs, linkages, interest groups, retail sites, and other educational venues, can provide ways to share information about internship programs.

FREESTANDING LACTATION COURSE WITH INTERNSHIP

Some freestanding courses taught by independent educators offer clinical internships to students. Lactation Education Resources (LER) (2012) is an example of this arrangement. The program has agreements with 12 hospitals in the metropolitan District of Columbia area, with each hospital accepting two to three interns per year. Internships are open to Pathway 1 and Pathway 3 candidates working toward IBCLC certification. Interns complete their didactic training online at their convenience, and when the course work is 75% complete, they may begin in the clinical area. LER serves as the primary mentor and provides oversight for each intern. IBCLCs in the various hospitals assume responsibility for day-to-day supervision and teaching of the intern. Homework and case studies are graded by the primary clinical instructor. When possible, interns are offered additional experiences in a private practice setting.

ACADEMIC PROGRAM WITH INTERNSHIP

Lactation programs that qualify IBCLC candidates through Pathway 2 are offered through academic institutions and include a clinical internship component. Some are degree programs and others are certificate programs. Some provide clinical experiences locally and others connect students to sites in other communities.

Some academic institutions offer lactation programs through partnerships with lactation educators. A certificate program offered through University of California-San Diego (2012) is an example of this type of partnership. The program is housed within the university's extension service and taught by an IBCLC. The university collaborates with sites throughout the United States to provide clinical experiences, with clinical instruction time donated. Union Institute & University (2012) offers a degree program through a similar partnership. Students complete didactic work through the university and the Healthy Children Project. They must locate sources for their clinical experience.

A one-year residential program is open to graduate students of the School of Public Health at the University of North Carolina at Chapel Hill (2012). Students complete a two-semester didactic course, followed by a clinical practicum, with supervised clinical at local medical training centers. Birthingway College of Midwifery (2012) in Portland, Oregon, offers a two-year Associate Degree program, with the supervised clinical component completed at the college and sites within the community. Multi-level commitment is essential to the success of such programs on the part of the academic institution, birthing facilities, and clinical faculty.

HEALTHCARE SYSTEM-BASED INTERNSHIP PROGRAMS

Being part of a large healthcare system has its advantages. In contracting, there is more leverage when services can be provided at facilities across a wide geographic area. There is the potential to leverage the power of the volume of products and services purchased to get a better price. There is potential for best practices to be disseminated to different sites without having to recreate the wheel.

There are also drawbacks inherent in trying to steer a larger organization, with greater varieties of perspectives and histories, all in one direction without resorting to the lowest common denominator. Getting a team together for multisystem work can present daunting challenges in scheduling and logistics. There may be resistance if the perception is that one site is dictating how others should do things without their input, or that decisions are being made through many layers of bureaucracy separated from the immediate hands-on caregivers or clinical instructors. The shared governance model can help.

The Carolinas HealthCare System (2012) has multiple acute care facilities, many clinics, and many primary care practices in a physician network spread over a two state area. It is approximately the 10th largest healthcare system in the U.S. Several sites have historically done informal or sporadic provision of lactation clinical education and experience hours. One facility (Carolinas Medical Center-NorthEast, a 450-bed community hospital, with about 3000 births/year and about 300 babies cared for through the level 3 NICU each year) in Concord, North Carolina, has generous lactation coverage, with a stable staff of experienced IBCLCs and a strong reputation for the highest quality of care. Commitment from the facility administration allowed for the development of a formalized lactation internship program through the continuing education department of the College of Health Sciences (Cabarrus College of Health Sciences) located on the same campus. There is a vision of expanding this program to use other sites within the system, and to have all the background courses, as well as the lactation-specific didactic coursework, eventually available through this program.

Presbyterian Hospital (2012), which is part of the Novant Health system in Charlotte, North Carolina, has an internship program with the lactation consultant department coordinating clinical instruction in three hospital sites and a pediatric office. Interns are encouraged to begin the clinical internship within one year of the time they complete an approved lactation didactic course. The Clinical Competencies for IBCLC Practice guides applicants in acquiring and documenting their clinical hours. The internship program can accommodate as many as 25 interns at the same time. Interns work with multiple instructors at a variety of inpatient and outpatient settings.

Healthcare system-based programs have great potential for meeting the needs of lactation consultant interns. Collaboration between a healthcare system and an academic institution facilitates the merging of didactic coursework with clinical experience into one cohesive program. Clinical experiences can encompass other acute care hospitals and community health science education programs. With the availability of on-line instruction, the internship could remain centered at one location with other sites connecting into it. Such a centralized lactation clinical program would accommodate interns and clinical instructors at multiple sites.

CONSORTIUM OF CLINICAL INSTRUCTORS

Another creative method for meeting the need for clinical experience is to create a collaborative consortium to provide lactation clinical internships with IBCLCs at a variety of sites in a geographical area. The USLCA chapter, Pennsylvania Resource Organization for Lactation Consultants (2012) has developed a Mentoring Consortium. The program is designed to provide a lactation intern with clinical experience in a variety of practice settings, including hospital, outpatient, pediatric, and private practice settings. The Mentoring Consortium coordinates placement of the intern at these different sites. This is a relatively new program, and it has been encountering difficulties finalizing contracts with clinical sites, particularly hospitals. Because the consortium is run by a nonprofit professional association, rather than an educational or healthcare institution, it is being challenged to meet insurance coverage requirements of hospitals. It has also grappled with whether and how much to pay the clinical sites for intern placement, how much to charge the intern, and how to ensure effective clinical instruction. The consortium has enrolled two lactation interns in the program as it continues to explore solutions to challenges it encounters.

SUMMARY

Support from ILCA and its affiliates provide essential stepping stones for the development and dissemination of educational programs. Collaboration and negotiation helps educators meet IBCLE and LEAARC standards and move the process forward. Rich resources are available through study modules and conference sessions related to education of prospective and currently certified IBCLCs, discussion boards, special interest groups, committees, task forces, and publications such as this one.

The best advice that can be given to someone who is considering starting a clinical lactation internship program is to access these rich resources provided by the lactation consultant professional organization and talk with those who have practiced these skills, learned hard lessons, and sorted out what may or may not work. Then go for it!

Chapter 7

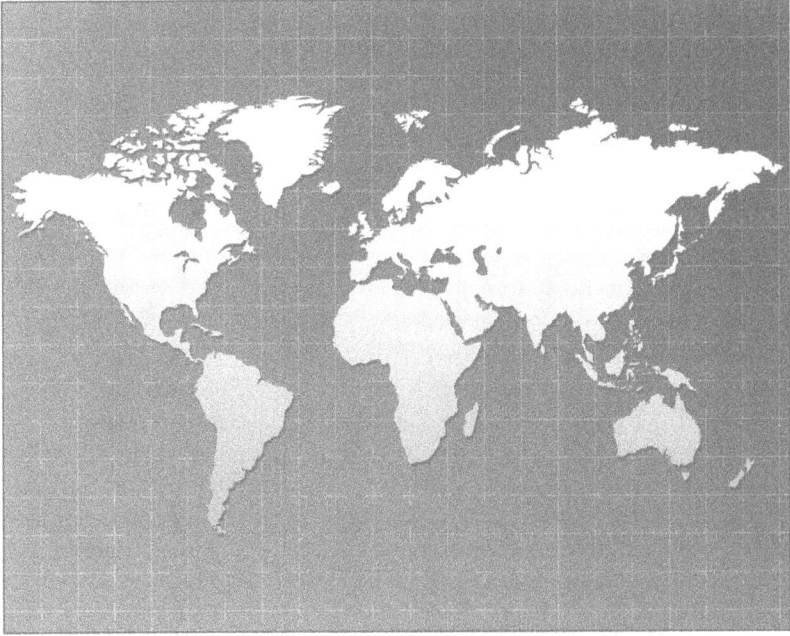

An International Perspective

There are differences in education requirements and preparation of IBCLCs in countries throughout the world. One universal challenge involves obtaining the variety of experiences needed. Hospital-based interns need the opportunity to work in a private practice or lactation clinics in order to acquire the experiences needed with later postpartum issues and older babies. For example, an intern who acquires all of her hours in an inpatient hospital setting, with no opportunity to see mothers and babies beyond the hospital stay, misses out on all the challenges that can arise after two to three days of life. In addition, an intern who is not allowed in the hospital setting, perhaps because she is not a licensed healthcare professional, will miss out on many of the early problems that can arise during the first days postpartum.

PRACTICES AROUND THE WORLD

While many descriptions and examples contained in this text are drawn from the U.S., the material is intended for a global audience. This chapter is devoted to country-specific practices around the world.

IN AUSTRALIA, the majority of IBCLCs come from a health professional background. IBCLCs work in hospitals, hospital-based lactation clinics, and in community-based child and maternal health clinics. Most large towns and cities also have IBCLCs in private practice. Clinical experience is gained during their employment, with alternative experiences being arranged by the IBCLC certificant.

IN BELGIUM, four universities offer education for lactation consultants, including both didactic learning and clinical instruction. Most IBCLCs are midwives and nurses, with a few pediatricians and general practitioners, and even fewer from mother-to-mother support. Most IBCLC certificants work in hospitals and home healthcare and learn clinical skills as part of their employment. Not many IBCLCs have their own private practice.

IN EGYPT, all the applicants to the IBLCE are physicians who must obtain 900 hours of lactation management to qualify to take the IBLCE exam. Most of the IBCLCs are pediatricians, and others are obstetricians or family physicians. The Egyptian Lactation Consultant's Association conducts a yearly 100-hour precertification lactation management program, of which at least 20% is clinical instruction (ELCA, 2012). Students bring interesting clinical cases to class, prepare case studies, and use the WHO breastfeeding counseling skills checklist, the breastfeeding observation job aid, and the feeding history-taking job aid (personal correspondence, Amal El Taweel, 12/9/11).

IN FRANCE, the Diplôme Inter Universitaire en Lactation Humaine et Allaitement Maternel (human lactation and maternal breastfeeding interuniversity diploma) is accessible to health professionals possessing the level of pediatric nurse or above (e.g., nurse, midwife, and physician). The IBCLC certification is not recognized by the French health ministry, so mothers cannot be reimbursed for a consultation unless it is declared a medical consultation. Hence, there is little room for independent IBCLCs who do not belong to a medical profession. As French university studies do not allow enrollment in a single course, the IBLCE requirement for basic educational background makes it unlikely that nonhealth professionals can become IBCLC certified. Health professional IBCLCs employed by a maternity unit, a NICU, or a Maternal and Infant Protection service are not able to teach interns during work due to insurance and responsibility reasons. Therefore, internship may be possible only in private practice.

IN ISRAEL, there is no country-wide requirement that to be an IBCLC you must be a medical professional. The ministry of health is working toward requiring all nurses to take a lactation course in order to work in a hospital. An issue for private practice IBCLCs who are clinical instructors mirrors the same concern in the United States: a client who is paying for a private consultation wants to see the IBCLC, not an intern (personal correspondence, Jessica Bilowitz, 12/22/11).

IN JAPAN, 80% of IBCLCs are midwives, 15% are medical doctors, and 5% are nurses or La Leche League Leaders without medical backgrounds. Most IBCLCs belong to the Japanese Association of Lactation Consultants (JALC), where continuing education is provided. JALC trains the facilitators who, as experienced IBCLCs, teach UNICEF/WHO's BFHI 20 hour course with clinical practice.

IN THE NETHERLANDS, a medical background is required to become an IBCLC with all experience obtained through that profession. Precertification education is provided by two schools which students attend for 24 days of instruction (one day per week for nine months). Many IBCLCs come from the profession "kraamverzorgenden," which is similar to a labor and postpartum doula in the U.S. She assists the midwife with the birth (30% of all births in the Netherlands are at home), and then comes to the home for seven to eight days after the birth for six to eight hours/day to assist with breastfeeding, bathing, and baby care, in addition to helping with the household and other children. IBCLCs who come from this profession do not have the medical background to work in a specialized area, such as a NICU (personal correspondence, Elly Krijnen, 12/9/11).

IN SPAIN, about 40% of IBCLCs are nurses, about 25% are pediatricians or midwives, and about 35% are support counselors without medical backgrounds. With the new IBLCE college subject requirement, mother support counselors will probably no longer be able to take the exam.

IN THAILAND, IBCLCs are primarily health professionals and are trained as part of the BFHI (Baby Friendly Hospital Initiative) staff training program. The clinical practice begins with an observation period, and then moves to being mentored and utilizing case studies as part of the clinical experience. There is a move towards making lactation management part of nursing and medical school academic programs (personal correspondence, Meena Sobsamai, 12/8/11).

IN THE UNITED KINGDOM, almost all IBCLC's employed by the National Health Service in a hospital or community setting are also healthcare professionals. The National Health Service is available to all and a private hospital for healthcare is not the 'norm.' Some IBCLC's are in private practice.

SUMMARY

Around the world, mothers and infants need help with breastfeeding challenges and families need education and support. Each country has unique patterns of preparing healthcare providers with the necessary professional education and skills. The overarching structures of IBLCE, ILCA and LEAARC provide for common concerns to be addressed. These organizations can promote standardization in the preparation of lactation consultants while allowing for the unique country-specific variety in ways to implement standards. With guidance and support from professional organizations, clinicians and educators throughout the world will have the fundamental resources to nurture the next generation of lactation consultant professionals.

Chapter 8

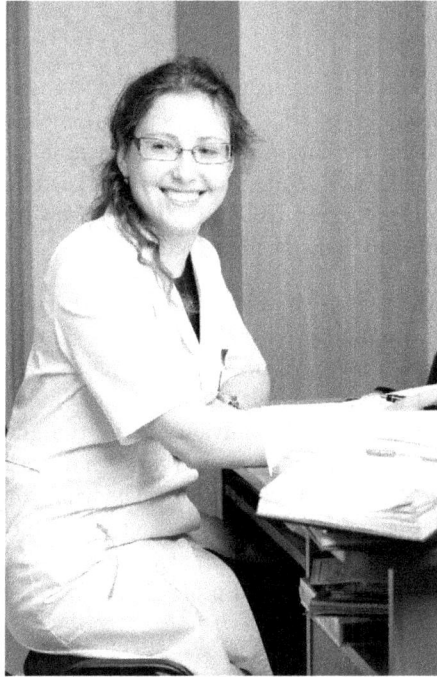

Concluding Thoughts

The focus of this text is teaching the next generation of IBCLCs. IBCLCs are a high stakes component for the future of preventative healthcare and health promotion. Thus, consideration of how the next generation of IBCLCs is to be developed and educated is worthwhile. The intentional development of future generations of lactation professionals is critical to the health of mothers and children. Healthcare professionals with specialized knowledge and skills in helping breastfeeding women can assist mothers to provide their babies a healthy start in life. Such specialized skills cannot be obtained without a foundation of thoughtful, supervised clinical instruction that produces skilled clinicians with the necessary practical knowledge and insights to provide optimal care.

In the short period of time since the formation of the profession in 1985, available knowledge and evidence-based practice has expanded dramatically. Avenues for education in lactation and supervised acquisition of clinical skills continue to evolve. The current climate for the professional development of

IBCLCs lacks a focused, intentional, standardized plan for preparing the next generation of clinical professionals. The profession needs a predictable, planned, and formalized structure for incorporating clinical education in the overall education of IBCLCs.

A VISION FOR THE FUTURE

Experienced IBCLCs who have acquired knowledge and skills are obligated to find ways to pass it on to the next generation. These wise mentors and educators help build for the future one intern at a time. Just as in any other profession, and especially in a young profession that is still evolving, there will be variability. Newly credentialed IBCLCs will bring new viewpoints and skills to build on the hard-won gains of their predecessors.

Imagine a future where there are clearly defined educational programs that provide consistent, comprehensive preparation in all domains: knowledge, psychomotor, and affective. Goal-directed individuals will see a clear path toward preparation to practice lactation consulting. Skilled guidance will be widely available from experienced individuals who can effectively help them learn and develop skills—both in person and through distance supervision with the use of technology. The IBCLC credential will be synonymous with "lactation consultant" and will denote the rigorous preparation for the profession, just as RN does for nurses and MD does for physicians. It will be clear to members of the public that IBCLCs are trusted professionals who can help them reach their breastfeeding goals.

IMPACT OF THE IBCLC

The structured preparation of IBCLCs will legitimize the profession and lead the way toward recognition of lactation consultancy by the Bureau of Professions in the United States and similar authorities around the world. As the professional authorities in lactation, IBCLCs will have an impact in all areas that touch the lives of breastfeeding families.

FOR PARENTS: IBCLCs will be clearly identified as the allied health professionals who are qualified to assist mothers and children with breastfeeding challenges. Parents will recognize the IBCLC as the healthcare professional who has the requisite knowledge and skills to provide clinical care services and help solve problems. Parents will be assured that their helpers are highly qualified because of the IBCLC credential.

FOR THE COMMUNITY: Those in the community who promote and support breastfeeding will recognize the IBCLC credential as assurance that the person has the necessary knowledge and skills to provide safe, effective, and helpful care.

FOR COLLEAGUES: Other healthcare providers and community-based breastfeeding supporters will recognize that they can rely on the IBCLC credential to denote those who have the background and capabilities to warrant referring parents to them.

FOR THE HEALTHCARE SYSTEM: Employers will recognize the value of IBCLCs and the need to employ them as the healthcare professionals in their facilities who render care to breastfeeding mothers and children. Recognizing the importance of this care, facilities will employ sufficient numbers of IBCLCs to provide the necessary level of care.

FOR THE PROFESSION: The lactation consultant profession will consist of IBCLCs who possess the necessary skills and knowledge and who obtain employment in the field in increasing numbers. IBCLCs can financially support themselves while practicing in a rewarding and challenging field, as respected colleagues in collaboration with other professionals on the healthcare team.

PASSING THE TORCH

Experienced IBCLCs are critical to the profession moving in this direction. Talented, knowledgeable, and experienced individuals with vision can work collaboratively through professional organizations, such as ILCA, LEAARC and IBLCE. Their joint efforts will protect consumers, advance the profession, and increase the likelihood that breastfeeding, with all its health protections and social benefits, becomes an achievable norm worldwide. With well-designed internships, experienced IBCLCs can be the leaders and teachers in this profession, with hope and action going hand-in-hand to advance lactation consulting into a future that is brighter for having footsteps to follow from esteemed colleagues who are no longer with us, but who showed us how to do this.

Appendices

Appendix 1

Planning Documents

INTERNSHIP PLANNING WORKSHEET

CLINICAL INSTRUCTOR APPLICATION

CLINICAL INSTRUCTOR/INTERN CONTRACT

CLINICAL SITE MEMORANDUM OF UNDERSTANDING

EDUCATIONAL CONFERENCES

EDUCATIONAL RECORDS

The forms in this section were developed for use in existing lactation programs. They were included to give people ideas for creating their own forms. These forms may be adapted for use in new programs as long as credit is given to the originating person/institution.

NUTS AND BOLTS OF PLANNING CLINICAL EXPERIENCE IN LACTATION

Phyllis Kombol, RNC, MSN, IBCLC, RLC

Activity 1: Consider and record your top 2 motivations for wanting to provide a program of lactation clinical experiences.

1.

2.

Activity 2: Make a list of your stakeholders (plan to meet with them individually and/or as a group).

Activity 3: Identify at least 3 champions/early adopters.
1.

2.

3.

Activity 4: Record at least 3 barriers/detractors; come back to reflect on their legitimacy/impact.
1.

2.

3.

Activity 5: Make a table listing potential clinical instructors. You and the clinical instructor rate each category as: 1=has potential, 2=adequate, 3=can do independently.

Instructor's name	Qualification/experience		Motivation		Teaching skills	
	Your eval	Instructor eval	Your eval	Instructor eval	Your eval	Instructor eval

Activity 6: Consider "who are our potential interns?" Make some notes about their resources/background/motivation.

Who	
Resources	
Background	
Motivation	

Activity 7: Evaluate your numbers/variety of patients. Go back later and consider in relation to IBLCE's exam blueprint re: time/topics.

How many couplets do you see in a day/month?	
What is their age range?	
How much variety in lactation issues do they represent?	

Activity 8: Review the three IBLCE pathways and determine which one(s) you will offer.

Activity 9: Rate your (group) readiness. If not ready, list the steps to getting ready with a timeline.

We're already doing this and just need to formalize the structure.

We're ready and almost everything is in place.

We're working on details.

We're in the design phase.

We're considering having a program.

Activity 10: Draft a basic business plan. Have at least one trusted colleague review it and ask you questions (develop 1-2 minute responses to the expected questions). Then have several of your stakeholders review the business plan and help you refine it before formally presenting it.

Activity 11: Draft your program description, goals, and objectives. Compare them to other models and review them as in the activity above.

Activity 12: Determine which of the college courses and continuing education topics could be co-requisites and which must be completed before entering the internship. Reflect on the pros and cons for each and consider where they can be obtained. List the sources you would recommend for obtaining lactation education and consider whether they are appropriate for everyone.

Pre-requisites required before entering internship	
Co-requisites completed during internship	
Pros and cons of having them completed before or during the internship	
Where can each be obtained?	
Lactation specific education hours: Sources you recommend Would a source be appropriate for everyone? Why or why not?	

Activity 13: Look at examples and design your own checklists that are specific to your site/program.

Activity 14: List 2 places people who complete your program are likely to get a job. Consider how well your program will prepare them for those specific sites...adjust.
1.

2.

Activity 15: List 3 other sites that could be part of your program.
1.

2.

3.

Activity 16: Continually review your program design, business plan, and other elements of your program and revise as necessary.

CLINICAL INSTRUCTOR APPLICATION FOR LACTATION CONSULTANT INTERNSHIP

Personal data

Name		Credentials

Street Address	City	State/Province	Postal Code	Country

Home Phone with Area Code	Work Phone with Area Code	Fax with Area Code

E-mail Address

Professional references
Provide the names of three individuals who can provide recommendations regarding your professional capabilities.

Name	Title/Position	Address	Phone number

Name	Title/Position	Address	Phone number

Name	Title/Position	Address	Phone number

Educational background

High School	Location	Year graduated		

College	Location	Dates attended	Degree Major	Number of Credits

Other	Location	Dates attended	Degree Major	Number of Credits

Lactation education

Title of lactation course	Course provider	Provider phone number	Date completed

Title of clinical instructor course	Course provider	Provider phone number	Date completed

Certification and licensure

Date of original IBCLC certification	Dates of IBCLC recertification

If you are a health care professional, please list all states in which you are licensed to practice. Attach a copy of the license from the state in which you currently reside.

Work/employment history
List employment history, beginning with the most recent.

Title	Length of service	Average hours per week	Average dyads seen per week

Employer	Supervisor	Phone	Address

Responsibilities:

Title	Length of service	Average hours per week	Average dyads seen per week

Employer	Supervisor	Phone	Address

Responsibilities:

Title	Length of service	Average hours per week	Average dyads seen per week

Employer	Supervisor	Phone	Address

Responsibilities:

Teaching experience
Describe any teaching experience in each of the following areas:

1. Breastfeeding classes for mothers

2. Inservices on breastfeeding for health professionals

3. Workshops for lactation consultants

4. Presenting at conferences

5. Clinical instructor positions

6. Other

Continuing education related to breastfeeding and lactation management
List and attach copies of certificates of attendance for continuing education for the previous five years.

Dates	Contact Hours	Title	Provider
Dates	Contact Hours	Title	Provider
Dates	Contact Hours	Title	Provider
Dates	Contact Hours	Title	Provider
Dates	Contact Hours	Title	Provider
Dates	Contact Hours	Title	Provider

Reference materials including periodicals
List five references you most frequently use in your reference library.

1.
2.
3.
4.
5.

Please respond to the questions below.
Attach additional paper as needed.

1. Have you personally received any funding from artificial baby milk companies? ___ No ___Yes ___ Unsure

   If yes, when and for what?

   Are you willing to reject such funding during your employment?   ___ No ___Yes

2. With what main site(s) do you have an agreement to provide clinical experiences to the Lactation Consultant Intern? Describe the setting, approximate number of dyads, and conditions frequently encountered at each site.

3. With which off-site areas do you have an agreement to provide experiences to the Lactation Consultant Intern? Describe the sites, the contact person, and the experiences provided at each site. Describe your expected involvement with off-site experiences.

4. Which experiences will the Lactation Consultant Intern be responsible for obtaining on her own?

5. Why do you think you will make a good clinical instructor?

6. What do you think will be the most challenging part of being a clinical instructor?

7. How will you restructure your present practice to accommodate teaching responsibilities with interns?

Please sign below
Your signature below indicates that all information provided in this application is truthful to the best of your knowledge.

_____   _____
Applicant Signature   Date

SAMPLE INTERNSHIP CONTRACT

Between Clinical Instructor (CI) and Lactation Consultant Intern (LCI)

The following is a contract between the clinical instructor (CI) *[insert CI name]* and lactation consultant intern (LCI)) *[insert LCI name]*, executed on this day of *[insert date]* for the CI to provide services as a Clinical Instructor to the LCI in pursuit of lactation consultancy clinical hours.

The principle site of this supervised clinical experience will be at: *[insert address of hospital or clinic]*.

This contract covers the program described in **Appendix A** which is attached to this contract. This program is to begin on *[insert date]* and will end on *[insert date]*.

The fee for this service will be *[insert amount]* to be paid by *[insert date]* or in installments of *[insert amount]* to be paid on the following dates: *[insert date]*, *[insert date]*, *[insert date]*.

Clinical Instructor Responsibilities:

1. The CI will provide the clinical experiences as described in Appendix B at the site so noted above or at the following site(s): *[insert address(es)]*.

2. The CI will assist the LCI in obtaining clinical experiences as outlined in *Clinical Experiences in Lactation: A Blueprint for Success (Blueprints)* at the off-site campuses listed in Appendix C.

3. The CI will review and grade written work completed by the LCI within *[insert number]* working days of submission.

4. The CI will be available by telephone and in person during daily business hours to the LCI when the LCI is at off campus sites.

5. The CI will notify the LCI of all conferences and evaluations at least *[insert number]* days ahead of time.

6. The CI will schedule all the conferences listed in Appendix E with the LCI before the end of the program.

7. The CI will seek out situations that will provide the LCI with beneficial learning experiences.

8. The CI will provide appropriate guidance and counseling during supervised clinical hours and during scheduled evaluations.

9. The CI will review the LCI's log and records of experiences weekly.

Lactation Consultant Intern Responsibilities:

1. The LCI will abide by the rules, regulations, policies and procedures of the institutions and sites where any experiences are obtained.

2. The LCI will be totally and personally responsible for arranging off-site clinical experiences as outlined in Blueprints and listed in Appendix D.

3. The LCI will submit written work to the CI within *[insert number]* working days.

4. The LCI will submit all written work neatly and in the following format: *[insert description]*.

5. The LCI will follow the dress code described in the Intern orientation.

6. The LCI will follow the policy for calling in absent or ill as described in the Intern orientation.

7. The LCI will actively seek out beneficial learning experiences.

8. The LCI will maintain a professional appearance and demeanor at all times and on all sites.

_____   _____
Clinical Instructor   Date

_____   _____
Lactation Consultant Intern   Date

Attachments: Appendix A
                Appendix B
                Appendix C
                Appendix D
                Appendix E

Internship Contract Appendices

APPENDIX A — Describe in detail the program that will be provided for the Intern.

Example: *The program will consist of [insert number] supervised clinical hours.*

APPENDIX B — Describe in detail the expected clinical experiences to be obtained and at which sites.

Example: *All experiences which are hospital based or outpatient lactation clinic based will take place at the home site listed on this contract with the exception of the NICU experience for which [insert name of facility] will be utilized.*

APPENDIX C — List and describe in detail which off site experience the Clinical Instructor will assist the Intern in obtaining.

Example: *Pediatric office experience at [insert name of pediatric practice]*
WIC/Public Health at [insert name and location of clinic]
Two hospitals maternity units at [insert names of hospitals]

APPENDIX D — List the off site experiences that the Intern will have full responsibility for obtaining.

Example: *Observing and teaching breastfeeding classes*
Observing childbirth classes
Attending mother to mother support group

APPENDIX E — List all education/discussion conferences to be held during the Intern's program.

Example: *Conferences which are detailed in the syllabus. The Clinical Instructor may add additional conferences that she intends to have with the Intern.*

SAMPLE MEMORANDUM OF UNDERSTANDING FOR CLINICAL AFFILIATION

between
[insert name of Hospital]
and
[insert name of Educator]

THIS AFFILIATION AGREEMENT is entered into by and between *[insert name of Hospital* (hereinafter "Hospital"), a health care institution in the State of *[insert state]* and *[insert name of Educator]* (hereinafter "Educator"), an educational institution in the State of *[insert state]*.

WITNESSETH:

WHEREAS, Educator desires to provide educational experiences to its Students enrolled in its Lactation Consultant Clinical Internship Program; and

WHEREAS, Hospital is willing to make available its facilities to said Educator, Faculty, and Students for educational training and clinical experiences which will necessarily include some activities and tasks performed by Students in learning the techniques of the Program,

NOW, THEREFORE, in consideration of the mutual covenants contained herein, the parties agree as follows:

I.   DEFINITIONS

1.1   Course. The specific Course within which the Student is currently enrolled to complete Program requirements.

1.2   Educational Experiences. Those clinical/educational activities taking place at Hospital leading to satisfaction of Course requirements.

1.3   Faculty. Qualified Educator personnel assigned as the responsible Faculty or the clinical instructor for Students participating in Educational Experiences at Hospital.

1.4   Patients. Any persons provided care, facilities or services, directly or indirectly, by or through Hospital or related organization.

1.5   Policies of Hospital. The Bylaws and rules of Hospital, the Bylaws and rules of the Medical Staff as approved by the Board, rules and regulations of the Department and other established policies, practices and procedures of Hospital.

1.6   President. The person holding the position currently titled President of Hospital or other such title as may hereinafter be adopted to describe the Executive of Hospital exercising overall authority with respect to the operation and management of Hospital.

II.   THE HOSPITAL SHALL:

2.1   Accept Educator's Students for which Student placements have been reviewed, planned and arranged for Educational Experiences by Educator. The number of Students eligible to participate in Education Experience will be mutually determined by agreement of both parties and may be altered by mutual agreement.

2.2   Make available those Educational Experiences and training agreed upon.

2.3   Arrange for an orientation program for the purpose of familiarizing the Students with Hospital's philosophy, policies and procedures for providing care, with its Patients, physical facilities, and such other aspects as are pertinent to Educational Experience of Students.

2.4   Provide conference and classroom space within Hospital facilities, as available, pursuant to mutually arranged schedules of use.

2.5 Provide necessary emergency care to the Students in the event of sudden illness or injury occurring at Hospital; the costs of such care to be the responsibility of the Student.

III. THE EDUCATOR SHALL:

3.1 Have the authority and responsibility for the Course and Program, including curriculum development, appointment of qualified Faculty to supervise Students, evaluation of Educational Experience, assignment of Students, and maintenance of educational standards.

3.2 Perform its responsibilities and obligations under this Agreement consistent with Hospital Policies and Procedures.

3.3 Provide, at least one (1) month prior to the start of any semester for which Students are to be placed under this Agreement, the anticipated number of Students, the proposed schedule planned, and the kind of Educational Experiences and activities desired.

3.4 Assign only Students believed to be in good health at the time of reporting for their Educational Experience, which includes a negative skin test for tuberculosis, and proof of immunization or natural history of mumps, rubella, and rubeola.

3.5 Educator agrees to require that its Students obtain and maintain, prior to the performance of this Agreement, appropriate infectious materials training which includes exposure to blood borne pathogens, infectious waste handling, preventing transmission of tuberculosis and the use of universal precautions as required by state and federal law, and any other training as required by the hospital.

3.6 Instruct Students on their responsibility for respecting the confidential and privileged nature of information which may come to their attention in regard to Patient medical records and other Hospital information. Hospital shall retain the responsibility for selection of Patient to be involved in training assignments with any Student, it being agreed that Hospital reserves the right to except any Patient from initial or continued involvement in program activities at Hospital.

IV. THE PARTIES AGREE:

4.1 Hospital and Educator shall maintain good communication between institutions and shall confer on plans, problems and changes related to the Educational Experiences of the Students.

4.2 Hospital shall notify Educator when any Student is determined by Hospital to be unacceptable for reasons of health, performance, or other causes which could interfere with Hospital operation or quality of patient care, and that upon receiving such notification, Educator shall withdraw any Student from assignment at Hospital.

4.3 Neither party, in performing its responsibilities and obligations under this Agreement, will discriminate against any person because of said person's race, creed, religion, national origin, sex or age.

V. INDEMNIFICATION

5.1 Educator shall indemnify and hold harmless Hospital from any damages Hospital may suffer as a result of claims, demands, losses, costs, or judgments arising out of the acts or omissions, of Educator, its Faculty, its clinical instructors, its Students, or agents, in the performance of obligations under this Agreement.

5.2 Hospital shall use its best efforts to give to Educator notice in writing within sixty (60) days after receiving any such claims made against Hospital, or after it has knowledge of any other damage, loss or expense threatened or incurred in regard to Hospital resulting from the above acts or omissions.

VI. COMPENSATION

6.1 This Agreement does not contemplate the payment of any fee or remuneration by either part due to the other, but is intended to jointly benefit both parties by improving the education and professional preparation of the Students.

6.2   Neither the Hospital nor the Educator shall at any time be held responsible for any compensation arrangements between the party of the clinical instructor and the lactation intern.

VII.   TERM AND TERMINATION

7.1   Term. The term of this Agreement shall be for one (1) year commencing on *[insert date]* and terminating on *[insert date]*.

    7.1.1   Renewal. This Agreement may be renewed for successive years upon mutual written approval.

7.2   Termination. This Agreement may be terminated as follows:

    7.2.1   Termination by Agreement. In the event Hospital and Educator shall mutually agree in writing, this Agreement may be terminated on terms and date stipulated therein.

    7.2.2   Early Termination. This Agreement may be terminated by either party with or without cause by delivering a written notice of termination to the other party at least thirty (30) days prior to such early termination.

7.3   Effect of Termination. All Students enrolled in the Program at the time notice of terminations is given shall be permitted to complete the Program until all required Educational Experiences have been offered to Students then enrolled. However, no other Students shall be placed at Hospital for Educational Experiences after the termination date or notice of termination date, whichever is sooner.

VIII.   STATUS OF PARTIES

8.1   In performing the services as contemplated hereunder, Hospital and Educator agree that Educator, Faculty and Students are acting as independent contractors and not as the agents or employees of Hospital. As appropriate, Educator and Faculty agree to pay, as they become due, all federal and state income taxes, as well as other taxes, including self-employment taxes due and payable on the compensation paid to the Faculty by Student and to indemnify and hold Hospital harmless from any and all taxes, penalties or interest which might arise by Faculty's failure to do so. This provision shall survive the termination of this agreement.

8.2   No Student in the Program will be deemed to be an employee of Hospital nor will Hospital be libel for the payment of any wage, salary or compensation of any kind for service provided by the Student. Further, no Student will be covered under Hospital's worker's compensation, social security or unemployment compensation programs.

8.3   The Student will, to the extent required by Hospital, maintain proof of health records, required insurances and progress toward educational goals.

IX.   GENERAL PROVISIONS

9.1   Assignment. Assignment of the Agreement or the rights or obligations hereunder shall be invalid without specific written consent of the other party herein, except that this Agreement may be assigned by Hospital without the written approval of Educator to any successor entity operating the facility now operated by Hospital or to a related or affiliated organization.

9.2   Waiver of Breach. The waiver by either party of a breach or violation of any provision of this Agreement shall not operate as nor be construed to be, a waiver of any subsequent breach hereof.

9.3   Governing Law. This Agreement shall be construed and governed by the laws of the state in which the Hospital resides.

9.4   Amendments. This Agreement may be amended only by an instrument in writing signed by the parties hereto.

9.5 <u>Notices</u>. Notices or communications herein required or permitted shall be given the respective parties by registered or certified mail (said notice being deemed given as of the date of mailing) or by hand delivered at the following address unless either party shall otherwise designate its new address by written notice:

> Educator
> Address
> City, State, Zip
>
> Hospital
> Address
> City, State, Zip

9.6 <u>Execution</u>. This Agreement and any amendments thereto shall be executed in duplicate copies on behalf of Hospital and Educator by an official of each, specifically authorized by its respective Board to perform such executions. Each duplicate copy shall be deemed an original, but both duplicate originals together constitute one and the same instrument.

X. EXECUTION

IN WITNESS WHEREOF, the duly authorized officers and representatives of Hospital and Educator have executed this Agreement on *[insert date]*.

HOSPITAL

By (signature): _____   Date_____

Printed name: _____

Title: _____

EDUCATOR

By (signature): _____   Date_____

Printed name: _____

Title: _____

EDUCATIONAL CONFERENCES

An Educational Conference is an instructional conference in which the clinical instructor discusses the items below. All items need to be discussed at some point during the internship. It will be most instructive to raise a topic when it is applicable to a situation encountered that day.

1. Maintaining professionalism in all interactions.

2. Avoiding, recognizing, and treating burnout.

3. Encouraging the mother to take responsibility for her actions; it is not the lactation consultant's fault if a mother chooses to stop breastfeeding.

4. Avoiding overloading mothers with information.

5. Recognizing when "enough is enough" with breastfeeding interventions attempted to resolve a problem.

6. Dealing with disbelieving or actively negative health care professionals.

7. Dealing with physicians whose practices compromise breastfeeding because of lack of awareness (for example, stopping breastfeeding for medications that are acceptable).

8. Developing business and professional relationships.

9. Avoiding giving away professional services over the telephone.

10. Following practices that provide protection from liability.

11. Seeing mothers and babies in person for problems rather than trying to resolve them over the phone.

12. Learning how to prioritize "battles" with other health care professionals.

13. Determining instances of "prescribing" in the context of the IBCLC's scope of practice.

14. Reviewing the IBCLC Standards of Practice and the importance of upholding them to the Intern and to the profession.

15. Reviewing the IBLCE Code of Professional Conduct.

16. Dealing with mothers who are difficult.

EDUCATIONAL RECORDS

PURPOSE

To ensure:
- quality and completeness of internship records
- a valid record of academic achievement
- security of intern records
- compliance with regulatory and accrediting agency requirements
- access to records by interns and faculty
- compliance with the Family Educational Rights & Privacy Act of 1974 (FERPA).

POLICY

1. Individual records for each intern ever enrolled in the Lactation Clinical Internship shall be maintained in Cabarrus College of Health Sciences Continuing Education office in locked, fire-resistant files and shall be available for use by Lactation Clinical Internship mentors and administrative staff only.
2. An intern who has a name change while enrolled is required to submit a legal evidence of such change immediately to the Chief Mentor who will forward the information to the College Continuing Education office.
3. An intern is required to notify the Chief Mentor (who will forward the information to the College office) immediately whenever there is a change of address or telephone number.
4. Interns may, upon request, be allowed to review their record. Such a review will be set-up according to the provisions of state and federal regulations. (see Access to Student Records Policies)
5. An "active" record contains the following information:
   a. application for admission
   b. authorizations for release of information
   c. evidence of US citizenship or I-551 card
   d. transcripts of records of previous educational experience
   e. correspondence
   f. medical record
   g. internship plan
   h. release of responsibility; confidentiality agreement
   i. record of orientation and completed ACE modules
   j. records of Blueprints workbook assignment completion
   k. any official documentation of intern performance/behavior as deemed appropriate by the Chief Mentor
   l. performance evaluations
   m. legal evidence of name change
6. At withdrawal or completion, the final summary of intern progress and the separation form are placed in the record and the record shall be closed.
7. A closed record contains documentation of completion and records of the individual's achievement in the program, immunization records and post-secondary transcripts, and will be kept for a period of six (6) years.
8. Components of interns' records not required in the closed record, as well as inactive admission files over six months old shall be disposed of by shredding.
9. Security and safe storage of records are ensured by: records of past and present interns for the past six years being stored in locked files in the Cabarrus College of Health Sciences office and backed up and stored off site daily; in addition, monthly back ups are stored off site in an undisclosed location, in an underground vault.
10. Upon written request of the intern and payment according to the published fee schedule, a copy of the completion record and other allowable components of the intern's record will be sent to the agency of choice.

REFERENCE

Family Educational Rights & Privacy Act of 1974 (FERPA) e-CFR 34.99
See the Authorization for Record Release form

8/10/2010

Used with permission Cabarrus College of Health Sciences, Concord, NC

Appendix 2

Application Documents

PROGRAM DESCRIPTION

APPLICATION CHECKLIST

APPLICATION FOR INTERNSHIP A

APPLICATION FOR INTERNSHIP B

INTERN VERIFICATION CHECKLIST

ENROLLMENT CHECKLIST PRECLINICAL

BACKGROUND AND SANCTIONS POLICY

BACKGROUND CHECK RELEASE

ACCEPTANCE LETTER

Carolinas Medical Center
NorthEast

Lactation Clinical Internship

Description of the Program

Lactation Clinical Internships are continuing education programs offered through Carolinas Medical Center-NorthEast Women's and Children's Services, in collaboration with Cabarrus College of Health Sciences, in Concord, North Carolina.

Purpose: These internships are designed to provide a formalized, structured program of mentored experiences in clinical lactation management and breastfeeding support. This is an intensive individualized experience-based program that can be tailored to a participant's learning needs. Participants are paired with mentors who are International Board Certified Lactation Consultants with at least 5 years of experience in a variety of clinical areas, and who have been recertified at least once.

Target Audience: This program is for individuals who are preparing for a job that includes providing clinical lactation management and breastfeeding support, or for individuals who want to improve their clinical lactation knowledge and skills. There are 3 courses. Two are specifically designed for people who are preparing for certification as a lactation consultant through IBLCE. The other course is designed for health care providers who wish to enhance their clinical lactation skills within their current health care qualification.

Timeline: The program length varies, depending on the individual participant's needs and which course is selected. Lactation Clinical Internships can be anywhere from 100 to 1000 hours in length, and may be completed over several weeks, or may extend over 1-2 years. For someone who is preparing for lactation consultant certification, and who has already completed a comprehensive lactation management didactic course, at least one year should be allowed for a full clinical internship before the annual July IBLCE exam.

[Link to IBLCE.org for exam eligibility requirements][Link to ILCA.org for lactation course listing]

7/20/10

Used with permission Cabarrus College of Health Sciences, Concord, NC

Date Received: _____

Course: _____

(This file will remain open for six months from the date received.)

Carolinas Medical Center
NorthEast

Lactation Clinical Internship Program
Application Checklist

NAME: _____

COURSE: _____

ADDRESS: _____

_____

PHONE: _____

ITEM	DATE REC'D
US Citizen? Yes _____ No _____ I-551 Card_____	
Application Fee ($50.00)	
Documentation of High School Graduation ___Diploma ___Final Transcript ___GED ____ College Transcript(s)	
Verification of Government Issued Photo ID and Social Security Card (visual)	
Letters of Reference: # 1 _____ # 2 _____ # 3_____	
Evidence of Courses (45 hrs of comprehensive lactation management – attach certificate(s) or transcript) Course Title: _____ Date: _____ Course Title: _____ Date: _____ Course Title: _____ Date: _____ Course Title: _____ Date: _____ Course Title: _____ Date: _____	
Healthcare Credentials: Indicate if current or inactive _____ (current or inactive) _____ (current or inactive) _____ (current or inactive)	
Essay submitted	
CHECKLIST COMPLETE Verified by Continuing Education:	
Signature:	Date:
Interview scheduled Interviewer name: _____ Date of interview: _____	
Signature:	Date:
STUDENT ACCEPTED YES NO	
Accepted by Women & Children's Services:	
Signature:	Date:

Used with Permission Cabarrus College of Health Sciences, Concord, NC

Carolinas Medical Center
NorthEast
Lactation Clinical Internship Program
Application

Print in ink or type all information below:

Name _____ Date of Birth _____
　　　(Last)　　　　(First)　　　(Middle/Maiden Name)　　　(Month/Day/Year)

Home Phone _____ Hospital Extension or Work Number _____

Cell Phone _____ Email Address _____

Name you prefer to be called _____ County of Residence _____

Mailing Address _____
　　　(Number and Street)　　　　(City)　　　(State)　　(Zip)

Gender	Ethnic Group/Race	
☐ Female	☐ American Indian	☐ Hispanic
☐ Male	☐ Asian	☐ Non-Resident Alien
	☐ Black	☐ White
	☐ Other: Please specify _____	

1. Are you a U.S. Citizen? **(If no, you must present a valid I-551 or Permanent Resident Card)** ☐ Yes ☐ No

2. Are you an employee of CMC-NE or one of its affiliates **OR** a CCHS student? ☐ Yes ☐ No

3. Are you a high school graduate? ☐ **Yes** ☐ No

4. Have you requested three (3) letters of reference to be sent to Cabarrus College of Health Sciences, attention Continuing Education? ☐ Yes ☐ No

5. Have you submitted documentation of a comprehensive lactation management course of at least 45 hours? ☐ Yes ☐ No

6. Have you submitted documentation of current and inactive healthcare credentials? ☐ Yes ☐ No

7. Have you submitted the required essay? ☐ **Yes** ☐ No

8. Have you ever been arrested, charged with or convicted of a criminal offense (either civilian or military) other than a minor traffic violation? ☐ Yes ☐ No
Are you now under pending investigation or charges of violation of criminal law? ☐ Yes ☐ No.
Have you ever been the subject of any adverse action(s) by any duly authorized sanctioning or disciplinary agency for either conduct based or performance based actions? ☐ Yes ☐ No
If yes, are any criminal charges pending against you at this time? ☐ Yes ☐ No
Please attach an explanation describing the circumstances and current status of any arrests, charges or convictions. Certain misdemeanors and/or felonies may make a participant ineligible for professional certification/licensure.

REFUND POLICY:
The $50 program application fee is NON-REFUNDABLE.

If you withdraw from the program on or before of the first scheduled day, we will send a full refund of tuition (less the $200 tuition deposit).
If you wish to withdraw prior to completing 10% of the program, we will refund 90% of the tuition paid beyond the $200 deposit.
If you wish to withdraw prior to completing 50% of the program, we will refund 50% of the tuition paid beyond the $200 deposit.
After completion of 50% of the program, interns will not be eligible for a refund.

I have read and understand the refund policy printed above.

_____　　_____
Signature　　　　　　　　　　**Date**

Used with Permission Cabarrus College of Health Sciences, Concord, NC

APPLICATION FOR LACTATION CONSULTANT INTERNSHIP

Personal data

Name		Credentials		

Street Address	City	State/Province	Postal Code	Country

Home Phone with Area Code	Work Phone with Area Code	Fax with Area Code

E-mail Address

Professional references
Provide the names of three individuals who can provide recommendations regarding your professional capabilities.

Name	Title/Position	Address	Phone number

Name	Title/Position	Address	Phone number

Name	Title/Position	Address	Phone number

Educational background

High School	Location	Year graduated		

College	Location	Dates attended	Degree Major	Number of Credits

Other	Location	Dates attended	Degree Major	Number of Credits

Lactation education

Title of lactation course	Course provider	Provider phone number	Date completed

Attach your certificate of completion.

Licensure

If you are a health care professional, please list all states in which you are licensed to practice. Attach a copy of the license from the state in which you currently reside.

Work/employment history
List employment history, beginning with the most recent.

Title		Length of service	Average hours per week

Employer	Supervisor	Phone	Address

Responsibilities:

Title		Length of service	Average hours per week

Employer	Supervisor	Phone	Address

Responsibilities:

Title		Length of service	Average hours per week

Employer	Supervisor	Phone	Address

Responsibilities:

Clinical experience in maternal/child health and breastfeeding
Describe contacts you have had with breastfeeding dyads in the previous three years.

Continuing education related to breastfeeding and lactation management
List and attach copies of certificates of attendance for continuing education for the previous three years.

Dates	Contact Hours	Title	Provider
Dates	Contact Hours	Title	Provider
Dates	Contact Hours	Title	Provider
Dates	Contact Hours	Title	Provider
Dates	Contact Hours	Title	Provider

Reference materials including periodicals
List five references you most frequently use in your reference library.

1.

2.

3.

4.

5.

Please respond to the questions below.
Attach additional paper as needed.

1. Do you have a copy of ILCA's Standards of Practice?

2. Do you have a copy of IBLCE's Code of Professional Conduct?

3. Why do you want to be a lactation consultant?

4. How do you respond when someone critiques your performance?

5. How do you respond when someone observes you clinically?

6. In what type of work situation do you see yourself practicing after becoming an IBCLC?

7. Life generates many simultaneous demands. How do you see yourself dealing with multiple demands as you try to meet your personal needs along with the written and clinical practice requirements of this program?

8. During this program, you may be required to be available for extended periods for clinical experiences, to do research and writing and to travel to clients' homes and to off-site experiences. What resources can you count on for support in meeting family, personal or other needs during this time?

9. What do you anticipate will be the most difficult aspect of your internship program?

Please sign below
Your signature below indicates that all information provided in this application is truthful to the best of your knowledge.

_____   _____
Applicant Signature   Date

INTERN VERIFICATION CHECKLIST

Intern Applicant   Date Approved

	Initial to Verify	Copy Received	Comments
Letters of reference			
Clinical Instructor's signature			
College transcripts			
Lactation course certificate			
Health care license			
Continuing ed certificates			
Malpractice insurance			
Criminal background check			
Hepatitis vaccination			
Rubella vaccination			
Tuberculosis test			
Drug screening			

Date Received: _____
(This file will remain open for 60 days from the date received.)

Carolinas Medical Center
NorthEast
Lactation Clinical Internship Program
Enrollment Checklist—Preclinical Screening

NAME: _____
COURSE: _____
ADDRESS: _____
_____
PHONE: _____

ITEM	DATE REC'D
Tuition Deposit ($200) Received	
Background Check Authorization Release Received	
Background Check Authorization Release sent to Human Resources	
Background Check Results Received and Reviewed	
Drug Screen Test Results (4 panel)	
Immunization Records: MMR: Titer _____ OR Dose 1_____ and Dose 2 _____ Hepatitis B: Titer _____ OR Dose 1_____ Dose 2 _____ Dose 3 _____ PPD Results (within last year?) _____ Tetanus (within last ten years) _____ Varicella: Titer _____ OR Dose 1_____ and Dose 2 _____	
ACE Modules Completed (attached transcript)	
American Heart Association Healthcare Provider CPR	
Malpractice Insurance (copy of certificate)	

CHECKLIST COMPLETE Verified by Continuing Education:		
Signature:	Date:	
File is sent to Program Coordinator	Date:	
NEO Express Scheduled _____ (date)		
Department Orientation Completed		
Intern receipt of Internship Handbook		
ID Badge & Parking Sticker Requested		
CERNER Training Scheduled _____ (date)		
ORIENTATION COMPLETE Verified by Women & Children's Services:		
Signature:	Date:	

Used with Permission Cabarrus College of Health Sciences, Concord, NC

BACKGROUND AND SANCTION CHECKS
(Lactation Clinical Interns)

PURPOSE
To conduct appropriate screening of applicants and monitoring of current interns to ensure a safe environment for staff, clients and interns at CMC-NorthEast.

POLICY
Potential Lactation Clinical Internship Participants are screened prior to official enrollment and as part of the determination of an accepted applicant's or intern's eligibility. This screening requires, but is not limited to, any or all of the following background and sanction checks:
- Social Security trace, criminal history, and North Carolina Sex Offender Registry
- Checks against duly authorized, licensing, disciplining and sanctioning authorities, including the Cumulative Sanction List of the Office of Inspector General.
- Continuing interns will be similarly investigated on a "for cause" basis.

Adverse reports could result in the denial of admission or non-continuance in the clinical program. All reasonable steps will be taken to verify that the information provided is accurate.

DEFINITIONS
Accepted Applicant – An individual who has applied for admission to the Lactation Clinical Internship and has been accepted to a specific course.
Conviction – The subject has either pled guilty or been found guilty by a judge or jury.
Falsification – Providing information contrary to that which is obtained in a background investigation (unless the background investigation is proven to be inaccurate) or omitting information and/or providing false, incomplete or misleading information.

PROCEDURE
1. All students offered admission to the Lactation Clinical Internship program will be required to complete and sign a release form to enable background and sanction checks to be conducted. Current employees of CMC-NorthEast may be exempted from the background and sanction checks if their background was searched upon initial employment or subsequent re-employment. Request for exemption shall be made by the employee upon admission utilizing the existing Background and Sanction Check form.
2. The Continuing Education office will be responsible for making the appropriate agency checks to determine if such individual has been the subject of any criminal conviction or adverse action, exclusion, debarment or other sanction; for each accepted applicant.
3. Documentation of the agency checks will be maintained in the individual's confidential file in the Continuing Education office. Applicants will be advised of any information obtained in the screening process, which could affect their admission and will be provided the opportunity to resolve any discrepancies or errors with the investigating vendor.
4. The application for admission to the Lactation Clinical Internship will include an attestation by the candidate relating to whether such candidate has been convicted of a crime or sanctioned by a duly authorized regulatory or enforcement agency of the government. Falsification of such information could be grounds for denial of admission. The following language shall appear on the admission application:
   a. Have you ever been convicted of a crime, either civilian or military, other than a minor traffic violation?
   b. Are you now under pending investigation or charges of violation of criminal law? If yes, explain.
   c. Have you ever been the subject of any adverse action(s) by any duly authorized sanctioning or disciplinary agency for either conduct-based or performance-based actions? If yes, explain.

5. The Continuing Education Director shall bring to the attention of the Chief Mentor and Nurse Manager of Lactation Services any individuals identified as having been sanctioned, charged or convicted of a criminal offense.

6. The Continuing Education Director will evaluate all accepted applicants who have been the subject of a criminal charge(s), conviction(s) or any adverse action for misconduct to determine if such charge(s), conviction(s) or misconduct should preclude final admission. Factors in determining such action include: level of seriousness of the charges or crime, the date of the charges/crime, the age of the person at the time of the incident, the nexus between the criminal conduct of the person and the activities of the academic program, the person's prison/jail probation, rehabilitation and employment records since the date a crime was committed.

7. The Lactation Clinical Internship Chief Mentor will take appropriate action regarding any individuals who are found to have been the subject of adverse actions by duly authorized legal or sanction authorities. In the case of an unacceptable background history, the offer of admission will be withdrawn and a refund of any tuition deposit or prepaid tuition will be made. There will be no refund of prior tuition payments for enrolled interns.

8. Convictions that will specifically preclude final acceptance for all students include, but are not limited to:
   a. A sex crime
   b. Exploitation of an endangered adult
   c. Failure to report battery, neglect, or exploitation of an endangered adult
   d. Murder
   e. Voluntary manslaughter
   f. Involuntary manslaughter within the previous seven (7) years**
   g. Battery within the past seven (7) years**
   h. A felony offense relating to controlled substances within the last seven (7) years**
   i. Abuse, exploitation, or neglect of a minor, child or dependent
   j. Failure to report the abuse of a minor, child or dependent
   k. Any act that, if it occurred at the organization, could compromise the safety or well-being of patients, employees, visitors, or volunteers of the organization.
   ** *Time frames are measured from the date of conviction.*
   In addition, the Lactation Clinical Internship will not accept any individual:
   l. Who has abused, neglected, or mistreated a patient or misappropriated a patient's property, as reflected in the state nurse aide registry, or
   m. Whose name appears in the N.C. Sex Offender Registry
   n. Any individual who has been convicted of a criminal offense related to health care or who is listed by a federal agency as debarred, excluded or otherwise ineligible for participation in any federally funded healthcare program, will be denied admission.

9. Enrolled interns must report, in writing, any criminal charge, conviction, or sanction to the Chief Mentor. For students in clinical courses, the notification must occur at least 24 hours prior to the next clinical class after the charges are filed or after the conviction or sanction occurs, or immediately if the charge/conviction/sanction occurs within 24 hours of the next clinical day. Failure to report a charge, conviction, or sanction could be grounds for immediate termination of participation in the intern's clinical activity.

10. The Continuing Education Director will attest to the Lactation Clinical Internship Chief Mentor and Nurse Manager of Lactation Services that interns participating in clinical activities have been screened and meet the criteria of this policy.

REFERENCE
CMC-NorthEast Human Resources Policy 2.31 (6/1/04).
7/20/10

Used with Permission Cabarrus College of Health Sciences, Concord, NC

Carolinas Medical Center
NorthEast

Background Check Release

In connection with my acceptance into and participation in the Clinical Internship in Lactation Program ("Internship") at Charlotte-Mecklenburg Hospital Authority dba Carolinas Medical Center - NorthEast (CMC-NorthEast), I understand that consumer or investigative consumer reports which may contain public record information, may be requested or made about me including criminal records, driving record, education, prior employer verification, workers compensation claims and others. Further, I understand that CMC-NorthEast will request information from various Federal, State and Local agencies regarding my past activities. I also understand that the information below regarding sex, race and date of birth is requested for the sole purpose of gathering the above information, and will not be used to discriminate against me in violation of any law. I further understand and acknowledge that such requests for information may be made by Cabarrus College of Health Sciences on behalf of CMC-NorthEast.

If negative information resulting in a change of my status with the Internship is contained in any report, I understand that I will be notified of such information by the Chief Mentor. I understand that information contained in the criminal background report might result in the termination of my Internship status. I also understand that any such termination may be appealed to the Lactation Nurse Manager and Women's and Children's Services Director. I understand that I am obligated to inform the Chief Mentor of any activities that may change the results of my criminal background report. I understand that I have a right to review the information that CMC-NorthEast and its designee receives in this criminal background investigation by written request. I understand that all reasonable efforts will be made by CMC-NorthEast to protect the confidentiality of this information.

I hereby release those individuals or companies from any liability or damage in providing such information. I hereby further release CMC-NorthEast and Cabarrus College of Health Sciences and its agents and employees from any and all claims, including but not limited to claims of defamation, invasion of privacy, wrongful termination, negligence or any other damages from or pertaining to the collection and/or dissemination of this information. I hereby authorize without reservation, any party or agency to furnish the above-referenced information.

I understand I have the right to make a request of the Consumer Reporting Agency, upon proper identification and the payment of any authorized fees, the information in its files on me at the time of my request. I further authorize ongoing procurement of the above-referenced reports at any time during my enrollment in the Internship.

_____   _____
Signature   Date

FOR IDENTIFICATION PURPOSES: PLEASE <u>PRINT</u> ALL INFORMATION CLEARLY

Last Name   First Name   Middle Name

Other Names: Maiden, Aliases, etc.:

Date of Birth: Month_____ Day_____ Year_____ Race: _____ Gender:_____

Social Security#:_____-_____-_____ Drivers License #: _____ State: _____

LIST ALL ADDRESSES FOR THE PAST SEVEN (7) YEARS STARTING WITH THE MOST RECENT/CURRENT

	Street	City	State	Zip	Dates (MM/YEAR)

1. _____ From: _____ To: _____

   _____

2. _____ From: _____ To: _____

   _____

3. _____ From: _____ To: _____

   _____

4. _____ From: _____ To: _____

   _____

5. _____ From: _____ To: _____

   _____

Cabarrus College of Health Sciences—Continuing Education
Carolinas Medical Center – NorthEast
920 Church Street, North
Concord, North Carolina 28025

7/19/2010
Used with permission Cabarrus College of Health Sciences, Concord, NC

Carolinas Medical Center
NorthEast

Lactation Clinical Internship Program

Date

Name
Address
City, State

Dear Name,

CONGRATULATIONS! You have been selected to enter the Lactation Clinical Internship program, a continuing education program offered through Women's and Children's Services at Carolinas Medical Center–NorthEast, in collaboration with Cabarrus College of Health Sciences. This is an intensive and individualized experience and we look forward to working with you to meet your goals.

Before you begin your scheduled clinical hours, you will need to complete your admissions file by submitting the following information denoted with an "X". Please note when the items are due.

-X- $200 non-refundable tuition deposit to secure a space in the program.
-X-   Consent for Background Check Release form (must be signed and returned by _____).
-X-   Official High School/College Transcripts (must be submitted by_____).
-X-   Copy of official CEU/CERP certificate or transcript showing completion of minimum 45 hours comprehensive lactation management course within the last 2 years. (must be submitted by_____).
-X-   Generic 4 Panel Drug Screen Form (must be submitted by _____). May be done by Employee Health.
-X-   Evidence of current PPD (must be within 12 months of first day of clinical and must be submitted by _____).
-X-   American Heart Association Healthcare Provider CPR certification is required (must be submitted by_____).
-X-   Proof of required immunizations listed on reenrollment checklist (must be submitted by _____).
-X-   Statement of Health Insurance form with copy of health insurance card attached (must be submitted by_____).

Included with this acceptance letter you will find important information that will help you with your program of study and planning your facility orientation. In the next few weeks you will also receive information about written work required prior to scheduling clinical hours. If you have any questions please contact the Continuing Education Coordinator, Janet Wright, RN, MSN, BC, at 704-403-3203 or the Lactation Clinical Internship Program Chief Mentor, Phyllis Kombol, RNC, MSN, IBCLC, RLC at 704-403-1186.

Again, congratulations and we wish you the best as you pursue your educational goals. Welcome!

Sincerely,
Phyllis Kombol, RNC, MSN, IBCLC, RLC
Carolinas Medical Center - NorthEast
Lactation Clinical Internship Program Chief Mentor

7/20/10

Used with permission Cabarrus College of Health Sciences, Concord, NC

Appendix 3

Orientation Documents

ORIENTATION CHECK-LIST

DRESS CODE

HEALTH POLICY

ALCOHOL AND DRUG ABUSE POLICY

DISCIPLINARY HEARING

WITHDRAWAL, SUSPENSION AND DISMISSAL

HANDBOOK TABLE OF CONTENTS

HANDBOOK ACKNOWLEDGMENT FORM

SYLLABUS

INTERN ORIENTATION CHECK LIST

	ORIENTATION ITEM	Date Completed	Intern Initials	Instructor Initials
1	Contract signed by both intern and clinical instructor			
2	How to use the *Blueprints* text or other required text(s)			
3	Working hours on campus			
4	Working hours off campus			
5	Dress code for on campus and off campus sites			
6	Picture ID			
7	Acceptable illness			
8	Calling in sick when scheduled on campus			
9	Calling in sick when scheduled off campus			
10	Physical layout of campus and parking facilities			
11	Introduction of other personnel and their job descriptions			
12	Location of resources			
13	Workplace safety, health and privacy regulations (e.g., OSHA and HIPPA) and fire, safety, emergency procedures			
14	Lunch and breaks, on campus and off campus			
15	Locker or drawer; intern's personal space			
16	Smoking breaks			
17	Daily routine involving mother/infant dyads			
18	Expectations of Intern during consults			
19	*Code* words or phrases			
20	How to address patients			
21	Beeper use			
22	Cell phone use			
23	When written work is expected			
24	Required format for written work			
25	When written work is to be returned to Intern			
26	Method of evaluation of written work			
27	Briefing conferences, timing and duration			
28	Intern's responsibilities for briefing conferences			
29	Debriefing conferences: timing and duration			
30	Intern's responsibilities for debriefing conferences			
31	List and dates of scheduled education conferences			
32	Daily paperwork and charting			
33	Evaluation process			

	ORIENTATION ITEM	Date Completed	Intern Initials	Instructor Initials
34	Evaluation forms			
35	Probation procedure			
36	Procedure for termination from the program			
37	Voluntary leave or withdrawal from the program			

Date Orientation Completed: _____

_____

Clinical Instructor's Signature

_____

Intern's Signature

Original to Clinical Instructor
Copy to Clinical Director
Copy to Intern

DRESS CODE

Lactation Clinical Interns are expected to follow the same standards as the Lactation Consultant staff in the clinical areas.

The following excerpt from the employee policy applies:

HR 5.01 – STANDARDS OF APPEARANCE

[Created: 8/1/88 Revised: 5/12/95, 6/1/96, 7/20/01, 9/9/05, 10/20/06, 7/9/07, 6/1/08 Reviewed: 6/1/08]

Summary

As professionals of Carolinas Healthcare System, we will present an image that reflects our commitment to quality care. Employees are expected to present themselves in accordance with the guidelines established for their profession and project a professional image through actions and appearance as required under the CHS Standards of Excellence.

Applicability

All employees of Carolinas HealthCare System.

Standards

This policy contains a set of core standards that applies to <u>all employees</u>. Standards are then further defined based on the following categories:

- [] Patient/Resident Care – Clinical
- [] Patient/Resident Care – Non-Clinical
- [] Support Business Units in Non-Patient/Resident Care Facilities

The following suggestions for dress and grooming provide guidelines. Management must communicate the expected Standards of Appearance as a part of the employee's departmental orientation.

Management may more clearly define work attire requirements in certain areas (ex., scrub color). Exceptions to this policy are permitted at the business unit level if approved by the accountable Senior VP, but must be put in writing and communicated to all employees with copies provided to the appropriate Human Resources Center.

Modifications may also be necessary for medical or religious accommodations reasons.

All Employees

- [] <u>Good judgment, which includes being well groomed and neat, is the main guideline to follow in dressing appropriately for work.</u>
- [] <u>Business dress is the default standard and is always appropriate.</u> When visiting another facility or business unit, follow or exceed their standards versus those of your home location.
- [] It is important you wear your photo ID badge at all times when on duty. The badge must be displayed at chest level or above with photo facing out so it is visible and readable to patients, patients' families, physicians and other employees. CHS Administrative Policy ADM 270.06 outlines restrictions on what may be placed on ID badges. For this and other information on ID badges, see CHS Photo Identification Policy, ADM 270.06, CHS Administrative Policy and Procedure Manual.
- [] If a uniform is required by the department, it will be worn according to unit/facility guidelines.
- [] All clothing will be clean, correctly sized, wrinkle free, and in good repair.
- [] Clothing should not expose bare mid-riffs or display cleavage.
- [] Undergarments must not be visible.
- [] Unless part of an approved uniform, hats will not be worn.
- [] Jewelry and other accessories must be conservative and not interfere with the performance of job duties or pose a safety hazard. Visible body piercings, other than earrings, are not allowed. Earrings are limited to two per ear and the top earring must be a post. Earrings should not exceed one and one-half inches in diameter and should not extend more than one and one-half inch below the bottom of the ear. Dental jewelry should not be worn while working.
- [] Tattoos should be completely covered or must be smaller than one inch in diameter and must not be offensive to our patients, visitors or other employees. Examples of offensive

tattoos include designs that are violent or threatening, sexual in nature, desecrate religious symbols, etc.

☐ Excellent personal hygiene is expected of all, including keeping hair and nails well groomed. Nail length will not interfere with job performance. Nail designs are not permitted and colors must be moderate. Extremes in hairstyle and color are not acceptable. Facial hair should be neatly trimmed if worn. Excessive use of colognes or perfumes must be avoided. Employees are not to have a recognizable odor of tobacco smoke when on duty.

☐ Dresses or skirts must be conservative in style and length, i.e., no more than one-two inches above the knee.

☐ Use of chewing gum is not permitted at any time in the presence of patients, visitors or guests or while on the telephone.

☐ Use of tobacco products including cigarettes, cigars, pipe tobacco, chewing tobacco, snuff, etc., is not allowed on CHS campuses or facilities or by employees during work time (HR 5.15, Tobacco-Free Workplace). Nicotine replacement products including gum, lozenges, nasal spray and inhalers may be used during work hours, but usage should be discrete and in accordance with physician and product manufacturer directions.

For examples of acceptable and unacceptable clothing choices, use the links within the sections below.

Patient/Resident Care Facilities

Clinical Employees

☐ Uniforms, shoes and socks must be of the color and construction designated by the respective department. Colored and/or patterned socks are permissible if they match the color scheme of the uniform and are not offensive in nature.

☐ Scrub suits, masks, shoe covers, and gloves are to be worn only in areas designated by department policy and only by those designated to wear them. Hospital scrubs are not to be worn off the premises. See CHS Administrative Policy ADM 270.05, System Provided Scrub Wear.

☐ Footwear for clinical areas must be appropriate for the work area. Safety will be a primary consideration when selecting footwear for work. Shoes must have a solid top surface and closed toes. Socks must be worn with Professional style Crocs.

☐ When caring for patients/residents, hair must be pulled away from the face and not hang into the patient care area.

☐ Nails must be clean, neat, trimmed and moderate in length. If polish is used, it must be one solid color and not chipped. Nail designs are not appropriate. Acrylic nail tips are not permitted in some work areas. If applicable, see Infection Control Policy # H71 (CMC) *Artificial Nails/Nail Length in the Facility* Policy and Clinical Practice Manuals (also in the Appendices section below) for additional restrictions.

☐ Patient and employee safety also dictates moderation in jewelry in clinical areas as hands must be adequately cleaned and numerous rings and bracelets may hinder safety. No jewelry is to dangle into the patient care space or hang over the patient in the delivery of care. See Appendix section for examples of **Clinical Attire**.

☐ When attending meetings or events out of the clinical environment, follow the standards for the area you are visiting. Example: When attending training sessions at the Airport Training Center (non-patient/resident care area), business casual is acceptable. [end of excerpt]

Lactation Clinical Internship interns are expected to adhere to the dress code of the facility to which they are assigned, and to present a professional appearance whenever they are in the clinical facilities. If the intern presents an unprofessional appearance in a clinical setting, the mentor `may send the intern off the clinical unit to correct deficiencies. For example, an intern who does not wear their nametag will be sent home to get it, or an intern who appears disheveled will be asked to correct their appearance to appear more professional. Time away from clinical to correct the deficiency will be counted as an unexcused absence.

7/20/10

Used with Permission Cabarrus College of Health Sciences, Concord, NC

HEALTH POLICY

PURPOSE: To provide information to interns regarding health issues that may affect them or patients

POLICY

1. Access: Emergency or urgent health care for Lactation Clinical Interns is accessible through CMC-NorthEast's Emergency Department and Cabarrus Urgent Care. Interns needing health services should follow the criteria as defined in personal insurance policies or contact the carrier for specific instructions. Interns needing non-urgent health services should contact their private physician or if none are available, report to Cabarrus Urgent Care.

2. Financial Responsibility: Interns are responsible for any fees or charges for medical care. Insurance may be applied, but it is the intern's responsibility to follow the criteria established by the carrier and present the appropriate insurance information at the time of service. CMC-NorthEast and Cabarrus College of Health Sciences assume no financial responsibility for referrals or for illnesses resulting from pre-existing conditions presented upon admission to the Lactation Clinical Internship program.

3. Pregnancy/Childbirth
   a. Should the intern become pregnant, she is required to consult a physician and continue prenatal care during her internship.
   b. When pregnancy is established, a conference should be held with the Chief Mentor to plan for the intern's maternity leave if it is anticipated to occur during the internship.

4. Physical Limitations
   a. In the event of physical injury, illness, or emotional illness that would limit clinical performance, the intern should notify the Chief Mentor and seek appropriate medical care and/or therapy. The intern must present a release from an appropriate healthcare provider to the Chief Mentor prior to returning to the clinical internship.
   b. In the event of surgery or hospitalization (including psychiatric in-patient or outpatient), the intern must present a medical release to the Chief Mentor prior to returning to clinical internship activities.
   c. In the event of behavioral difficulties (such as depression, marital and emotional problems, stress, chemical abuse, financial difficulties and other emotional problems) the intern may be referred to the appropriate professional for consultation and follow-up. The intern must present a medical release to the Chief Mentor prior to returning to internship activities.
   d. NOTE: Release must document intern's ability to perform at the physical and emotional standards required for the Lactation Clinical Internship.

5. Illness/Infectious Diseases: To protect the patients, co-workers, and the intern, the intern is expected to call in sick for any illness that is communicable, or any illness that results in the intern being unable to perform expected clinical activities. This call is expected to be at least 2 hours prior to the start of the clinical day, and may be by voice mail to the Lactation office 704-403-1186. An intern who has been diagnosed with an infectious and/or contagious disease must present a medical release to the Chief Mentor prior to returning to internship activities.

8/2010

Used with permission Cabarrus College of Health Sciences, Concord, NC

ALCOHOL AND DRUG ABUSE POLICY

PURPOSE
To provide a safe and productive drug-free work environment.

It is the policy of CMC-NorthEast that employees, students, or interns shall not use, possess, purchase, sell, transfer, distribute or manufacture any illegal drug at any time, or use or possess alcohol on the campus, clinical or fieldwork sites, or CMC-NorthEast premises. Nor shall any student, intern, or employee be under the influence of any illegal drug or alcohol while on the job, on CMC-NorthEast premises, operating a CMC-NorthEast vehicle, or engaged in College and CMC-NorthEast business. The policy includes employees who are on call. Any student, intern, or employee who observes behavior of any healthcare provider that is consistent with possible alcohol or substance abuse should report the behavior to the immediate instructor/mentor and/or supervisor. Whatever steps deemed necessary for the protection or safety of others should be taken.

PROCEDURES

Legal Drugs
Interns should be aware that many cough syrups and other over-the-counter liquid medications contain substantial amounts of alcohol. Use of these preparations is prohibited prior to or while conducting business on the CMC-NorthEast campus, clinical or fieldwork sites. Interns should inform their Chief Mentor if this type of cough syrup has been prescribed by a physician. A physician may consider a non-alcoholic alternative if he/she is made aware of the alcohol and drug abuse policy.

Legal drugs may also affect the safety of the intern, fellow employees/students or members of the public. Therefore, any intern who is taking any legal drug which the prescribing physician or pharmacist indicates might adversely affect the intern's ability to safely perform the functions of his or her duties as an intern must advise his or her Chief Mentor before reporting to clinical under such medication. If it is determined that such use adversely affects the intern's ability to safely perform the functions of his or her assignments or job, an excused absence may be granted during the period of treatment. If it is determined that such use does not pose a risk, the intern will be permitted to attend clinical. Improper use of "legal drugs" is prohibited and may result in disciplinary action. Prescription medication must be kept in its original container if such medication is taken on the CMC NorthEast campus, clinical/fieldwork sites.

Definitions
  A. **Illegal Drug** – any drug that is illegal under federal, state, or local law, or which has been illegally obtained, or for which a valid prescription is required and lacking, or any drug when used contrary to a valid prescription, its intended use, or the instructions of a licensed health care professional.
  B. **During Clinical** — includes all time during regular clinical hours, including breaks and rest periods, whether the person is on or away from CMC-NorthEast property, and further includes hours beyond regular class and working hours when an intern engaged in CMC-NorthEast business.
  C. **CMC-NorthEast Campus, Clinical or Fieldwork sites**— includes any location where the business of the CMC-NorthEast is being conducted by one or more interns, students, employees, or authorized representatives.
  D. **Positive Test Result** — the result of a test performed by an approved laboratory which shows that an intern has taken illegal drugs at any time, or that any intern was under the influence of alcohol during regular clinical hours, or while engaged in clinical/fieldwork or CMC-NorthEast business.

TESTING
  A. **Pre-enrollment Testing for Interns**
    1. It is the applicant's responsibility to obtain a standard four-panel urine drug screen not more than 30 days prior to the initial enrollment in any course with a clinical component. This may be done as part of the health screening at Employee Health. A urine test will be conducted to determine presence of amphetamines, cannabinoids, cocaine metabolites, and opiates.
    2. The results of the urine drug screen must be sent directly to the attention of the Cabarrus College of Health Sciences Continuing Education office from the testing facility.
    3. A negative urine drug screen is required for enrollment. A positive urine drug screen will result in the rejection of the applicant.
    4. Correspondence regarding rejection of admission will be remitted to the Chief Mentor.
    5. Should the applicant reapply, the applicant will be viewed as applicant status only and not as a readmission, since the applicant was not previously admitted.

  B. **Periodic Testing During Enrollment** The organization reserves the right to have interns undergo testing in the following situations:
    1. **After Charge or Arrest:** Any intern who has been charged with or arrested for a drug or alcohol-related crime, including DWI, may be required to undergo periodic drug testing. Interns are required to notify the Chief Mentor of any arrests related to drug and alcohol use.
       a. Interns — As soon as the Chief Mentor is aware of an arrest for drug use or possession, the intern will be required to submit to a urine drug test. If the test is positive, the intern will be subject to termination.
       b. Interns –The intern is suspended from clinical attendance until the legal matter is resolved. If convicted, the intern may be subject to termination.
    2. **Accidents or Unsafe Behavior:** Any intern involved in an on-the-job accident, and or on the campus accident resulting in more than an estimated $100 in damage to the CMC-NorthEast property, or conduct which constitutes a safety violation or nearly causes an accident may be subject to drug and alcohol testing.
    3. **Display of Impaired Behavior:** Whenever an intern displays unusual behavior which suggests that he or she may be under the influence of alcohol or drugs, such as but not limited to: slurred speech, imbalance, erratic behavior or other conduct which in the opinion of management suggests impairment, then such intern may be subject to drug and alcohol testing.
  C. As Required by North Carolina Law, any positive tests will be confirmed by a laboratory which has been certified by appropriate authorities to conduct such tests. Interns and applicants further have the right under North Carolina law to have any positive samples retested at the same or a different laboratory at their own expense.

D. The results of all tests shall remain confidential except as required to carry out required management actions and/or to notify appropriate professional licensing authorities.
E. All drug and alcohol tests, with the possible exception of pre-admission tests, may be performed without prior notification and will be carried out as soon as feasible upon management determination that criteria for testing are met. Such testing will be performed using accepted procedures assuring the accuracy of testing results, including the use of qualified testing personnel and certified testing laboratories and equipment. Such tests include urine testing, breath testing, saliva testing and blood testing to detect illegal drug use or impairment due to alcohol use. Impairment due to alcohol use is determined to be present with the equivalent of a blood alcohol concentration of 0.04 or higher. This is half the limit for driving while intoxicated under current North Carolina law.

PROCEDURE FOR TESTING

A. Interns suspected of being under the influence of drugs or alcohol should be removed from the clinical, fieldwork and/or work area immediately by the mentor, manager and/or supervisor.
B. The mentor, manager and/or administrative coordinator should observe the intern and document observations.
C. The intern should be given the opportunity to explain in writing his/her condition.
D. The mentor and/or manager shall accompany the intern to the Employee Health office.
E. Tests for breath or blood alcohol and urine tests for illegal drugs will be collected by the Employee Health personnel using chain of custody procedures. Tests will be sent to the reference lab for actual analysis.
F. Results for interns will be sent to the Continuing Education Director.
G. All paper work, i.e. consent form, Chain of Custody documents and results will be retained as part of the intern's records.
H. Interns tested for "for-cause" will be removed from clinical or fieldwork until the results of testing are available. If drug and alcohol tests are negative, the intern will be allowed to return to clinical. Any clinical work that is missed may need to be rescheduled at the discretion of the Chief Mentor.
I. Drugs for which interns are tested may include alcohol, cocaine, marijuana, phencyclidine, amphetamines, benzodiazepines, barbiturates, opiates, hallucinogens (such as LSD), depressants, stimulants or any other drug the use of which may lead to performance impairment, addiction, or other adverse consequences. Specific concern regarding the use of particular substances may lead to testing for such substances.
J. An intern who is screened under the "for cause" process and for which the test result indicated the presence of illegal drugs or abuse of legal drugs will be considered positive.

INSPECTION

Interns shall be required to submit to an inspection of their person and of their personal property located on the CMC-NorthEast premises or fieldwork sites, and/or whenever the mentor has reason to suspect that violations of this policy are occurring. Persons may be required to empty the contents of their clothing, purses, backpacks, and other personal containers and have their clinical or fieldwork site carefully inspected. Interns may also be required to permit inspection of their personal vehicles located on the campus or fieldwork site. Inspections under this paragraph shall be permitted only if authorized by the Nurse Manager of Lactation Services.

GROUNDS FOR TERMINATION

A. Interns will be subject to termination if they test positive for illegal use at any time or test positive for being under the influence of alcohol during regular clinical or fieldwork hours. Interns will be subject to termination if they possess, purchase, sell, transfer, distribute, manufacture, or consume illegal drugs or alcohol on the CMC-NorthEast premises or fieldwork sites or during any hours when business is being conducted.
B. Interns will be subject to termination if they refuse to submit to any required testing or inspections.
C. Persons engaged in out of class and/or off-the-job possession, transfer, manufacture, or distribution of illegal drugs shall be subject to termination.
D. An intern who in any way attempts to improperly alter the samples or result of a drug or alcohol test will be subject to termination.

REFERENCE
CMC-NorthEast (2002). *Human Resources Policy and Procedure Manual: Alcohol and Drug Abuse* (Policy No: 5.02)
CMC-NorthEast. *Human Resources Policy and Procedure Manual: Charges, Convictions or Sanctions* (Policy No: HR 5.30)
8/10/2010

DISCIPLINARY HEARING

PURPOSE

To define the process of the disciplinary hearing procedure in order that student rights be protected.

POLICY

The disciplinary hearing procedure to be followed where suspension or dismissal for other than academic reasons may result shall be as follows.

1. Each intern, against whom a complaint is received, shall be submitted a written notice, or statement of charges, signed by the Nurse Manager of Lactation Services, to inform the intern of the specific complaint against him or her. Such notice shall be sufficiently particular in stating facts so as to inform the intern of the nature of the alleged infraction. The notice shall specifically state the date, time, and place of the scheduled hearing, and shall list the names of each witness who will appear and testify at the hearing.

2. The hearing shall be held before the Nurse Manager of Lactation Services and Chief Mentor of the Lactation Clinical Internship, not sooner than twenty-four (24) hours or no later than ten working days after a complaint is received concerning any intern. All complaining witnesses and the intern against whom the complaint is made shall be present at the hearing. Neither the complaining witnesses nor the intern charged shall be entitled to representation by an attorney at the hearing. The intern charged shall be entitled to cross-examine all witnesses.

3. If the intern against whom the complaint is made does not appear at the hearing, the hearing shall be conducted in the absence of the intern.

4. The foregoing disciplinary hearing procedure shall apply only to those charges where written notices of the same may result in suspension or dismissal.

5. At the conclusion of the hearing, or within a reasonable time thereafter, the Nurse Manager of Lactation Services shall announce the decision in the case to the intern charged, and a written memorandum of findings shall be made a part of the record of the proceedings and a copy of the same shall be given to the intern charged.

6. If the intern charged is suspended, or dismissed, as a result of the final decision of the Nurse Manager of Lactation Services, then the intern may appeal the final decision to the Director of Women's and Children's Services.

7/20/10

Used with permission Cabarrus College of Health Sciences, Concord, NC

WITHDRAWAL, SUSPENSION, AND DISMISSAL

PURPOSE
To define procedures that will guide the Lactation Clinical Internship Mentor(s) and intern through the voluntary and involuntary withdrawal processes.

POLICY
Withdrawal may be:
1. Voluntary
   a. First, the intern must submit a letter of withdrawal to the Chief Mentor.
   b. An intern wishing to withdraw voluntarily should obtain the Withdrawal Form (see attachment), complete all parts of the form, and return the completed form to the College Continuing Education office.
   c. For withdrawal to be finalized, the intern's completed Withdrawal Form must be filed with their completion records at the College. The date the College office receives the completed Withdrawal Form is the official date of withdrawal.
2. Involuntary (Dismissal)
   a. An intern is expected to meet certain standards to remain in the Lactation Clinical Internship. If at any time it is the judgment of the Mentors and administration that an intern has failed to meet the academic, behavior, or health policies, the intern may be suspended or dismissed.
   b. An intern may be suspended for a specific period of time to allow time for fact-finding and decision-making regarding the incident in question. During a suspension, an intern will not be allowed to participate in any clinical activities.
   c. Any intern failing to meet required standards will not be allowed to progress in the program
   d. It shall be the duty of the Chief Mentor to communicate to the intern, and record any decision concerning the intern's status, which is then added to the intern's records at the College.
   e. The faculty and administration are committed to assisting each intern in every way possible to complete the program successfully, but are also responsible for dismissing the intern who:
      (1) does not meet clinical standards
      (2) is an unsafe practitioner in the clinical area
      (3) is dishonest
      (4) is absent excessively
      (5) fails to comply with professional behavior policies
      (6) fails to meet financial obligations
      (7) fails to comply with policies of the clinical facilities
      (8) presents physical and/or emotional problems that do not respond to appropriate treatment and/or counseling within a reasonable period of time
      (9) fails to submit to testing for alcohol or drugs.
   Some additional, but not all-inclusive reasons for dismissal are:
      (1) fraudulent marking or falsification of any record
      (2) removal without permission, or misuse of records or confidential information of any nature
      (3) engaging in any anti-social, criminal, dangerous, or violent activity
      (4) fighting or misconduct on clinical premises
      (5) obscene or offensive language or behavior in the clinical facilities, including sexual harassment
      (6) attending clinical while under apparent influence of alcohol, drugs, stimulants, or debilitating substances
      (7) selling, distributing, or giving unauthorized drugs or alcohol to students, employees, patients, or visitors
      (8) theft or misappropriation of CMC-NorthEast's, student's/intern's, employee's, patient's, or visitors' property, or removal of any such property from the premises without permission
      (9) tampering with, damaging, or using clinical facility property without permission
      (10) failure to report acts of dishonesty
      (11) noncompliance with corporate email policies
3. The decision concerning suspension, or dismissal for any reason shall be the responsibility of the Chief Mentor and Nurse Manager of Lactation Services.

REFERENCE
See the Withdrawal Form attached   7/20/10

Used with permission Cabarrus College of Health Sciences, Concord, NC

Carolinas Medical Center
NorthEast
Lactation Clinical Internship
INTERN WITHDRAWAL FORM

Instructions: To ensure that all obligations (Student to College and College to Student) have been fulfilled:
- ☐ Meet with Chief Mentor to complete the "Student" section
- ☐ Meet with the College/Continuing Education personnel re: financial eligibility for refund
- ☐ Meet with the Chief Mentor or College office secretary to return ID badge
- ☐ Submit the form to the College Continuing Education office

STUDENT Section:

Name | Date

Address

SS# | Home Phone | Work Phone | Cell Phone | Forwarding E-Mail Address

Program | Date of last class attended | Date enrolled | Chief Mentor

Reason for Withdrawal:
☐ Academic ☐ Medical ☐ Personal ☐ Financial ☐ Dismissal ☐ Other _____
Are you transferring to another college? ☐ Yes ☐ No   If yes, which college? _____

By signing above, I certify that all of the above information is true and correct. | Date

Chief Mentor's Signature | Date

FINANCIAL Section:

Financial: eligible for refund? ☐ Yes ☐ N/A | Student Account Cleared ☐ Yes ☐ No Explain:_____

Continuing Education Director Signature: | Date

COLLEGE OFFICE Section:

☐ ID Badge Returned (#_____) or ☐ $10 Badge Fee Paid | ☐ Parking Tickets Cleared | ☐ Library Clearance

College/Continuing Education Director Signature:

Date of Withdrawal:

Records Release Approval ☐ Yes ☐ No
Date:

Record closed by:
Date:

7/20/10

Used with permission Cabarrus College of Health Sciences, Concord, NC

Carolinas Medical Center
NorthEast

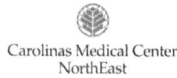

Lactation Clinical Internship
Participant Handbook

Table of Contents

Policies
> Alcohol and drug abuse policy
> Background and Sanctions checks
> Disciplinary hearing
> Dress code
> Educational records
> Enrollment of participants with disabilities
> Evaluations:
>> Evaluation of lactation interns
>>> Daily evaluation
>>> Monthly evaluation
>>> Final evaluation
>> Evaluation of mentors
>> Program evaluation by participant
> Health policy
> Withdrawal, suspension, dismissal (Withdrawal form attached)

Student handbook agreement form

7/24/10

Used with Permission Cabarrus College of Health Sciences, Concord, NC

Carolinas Medical Center
NorthEast

LACTACTION CLINICAL INTERNSHIP
HANDBOOK ACKNOWLEDGEMENT

I have read the material in the current Lactation Internship Handbook and understand it. As a Lactation Clinical Intern, I understand that I must comply with the policies contained in the Handbook to continue in the program. I understand that this Handbook is reviewed/revised every year, and changes will be reviewed with me when they occur.

I understand that all information regarding clients is strictly confidential, whether written in the hospital record or coming to my knowledge from being in the health care facility and I will not violate confidentiality. **I will not photocopy, download or otherwise record any clinical site record.**

I am aware of the inherent problems present in the clinical settings regarding lifting clients, communicable diseases that clients have, the potential for needle sticks, exposure to hazardous materials and radiation, etc. I am also aware that these hazards are always present and proper precautions must be taken at all times. I am aware that I must use standard precautions in caring for all clients.

Name (print): _____

Signed: _____

Date: _____

Please sign this form and return it to the Chief Mentor.

Lactation Clinical Internship Handbook
Adapted from CCHS Nursing Student Handbook
2010-2011
7/20/10

Used with Permission Cabarrus College of Health Sciences, Concord, NC

Carolinas Medical Center
NorthEast

Women's and Children's Services
In collaboration with
Cabarrus College of Health Sciences—Concord, NC

Lactation Clinical Internship Program

Course # 103 Full Lactation Clinical Internship

Syllabus—July 2010

Phyllis Kombol, RNC, MSN, IBCLC, RLC—Chief Mentor
Dawn Deinert, RN, IBCLC, RLC—Mentor
Eileen Black, RN, BSN, IBCLC, RLC—Mentor

Description of Course Content

This comprehensive lactation internship is intended to assist the participant to develop lactation clinical skills in all areas of clinical lactation practice: inpatient, outpatient, specialty units, community sites, office sites. This program is designed to meet the IBLCE's 500 hour supervised internship requirement for certification using Pathway 3. All areas of the IBLCE exam blueprint will be covered, and all areas of the IBLCE competency skills checklist will be mastered (see IBLCE skills competency checklist)

IBLCE exam candidates must get IBLCE approval for the internship as indicated in the Pathway 3 Guide, and must apply for IBLCE exam as indicated in the Exam Application Guide (see IBLCE.org). Mentors will be able to assist the candidates with this process.

Prerequisites

A comprehensive lactation management course of 45 or more clock hours must have been completed within the last 2 years. Participants must have lactation clinical internship chief mentor approval (interview and screening process). In addition, the participants accepted for this course will have successfully completed at least 75% of the didactic sheets on maternal and infant conditions from the workbook "Clinical Experience in Lactation: A Blueprint for Intenrship, 2nd edition" by Barger and Kutner (available through ILCA.org) before on-site clinical hours are scheduled to begin.

Credit

A certificate of completion will be awarded through the Continuing Education Department of Cabarrus College of Health Sciences at the completion of all course requirements.

Clinical Length

The course includes a minimum of 750 hours to be completed over approximately 1 year, including observation time. This course will meet the IBLCE Pathway 3 requirements of 500 hours of supervised practice.

Course Objectives

Participants will:

- Observe experienced IBCLCs in a variety of practice areas.
- Receive guidance through the process of increasing clinical skills.
- Independently perform all aspects of lactation consultant practice under the supervision of experienced IBCLC mentor(s).

Teaching Strategies

Initially the intern observes the experienced IBCLC, then increasing participation by the intern in lactation clinical care as described in the IBLCE Phases of Internship.

Student Learning Outcomes

Student Learning Outcomes

Upon completion of the experiences in this course, using the "Clinical Experience in Lactation: A Blueprint for Internship, 2nd edition" (2010) by Barger and Kutner, the participant will be able to: (the following objectives list used with permission of Barger and Kutner)

1. Verbalize understanding of the prenatal education available to pregnant women, and how breastfeeding information is presented throughout.
2. Teach a prenatal breastfeeding class as a part of a childbirth education series.
3. Teach a prenatal breastfeeding class as a stand-alone class
4. Verbalize understanding of the impact of medications and interventions used in the labor and birthing process on the breastfeeding dyad.
5. Increase ability to assist mothers and infants with the first feed in the birthing unit.
6. Develop adeptness at working with mothers and infants who exhibit common breastfeeding problems in the first three days of life.
7. Demonstrate appropriate use of breast pumps and alternative feeding methods for infants.
8. Develop a plan of care for breastfeeding infants in the NICU/SCN.
9. Verbalize understanding of how hospitalization of either mother or infant can impact the breastfeeding relationship.
10. List the types of breastfeeding problems and interventions that are commonly seen in an outpatient lactation clinic or private lactation consultant practice.
11. Verbalize understanding of how the breastfeeding dyad receives lactation help at the pediatric office.
12. Become adept at assisting mothers in using varying breastfeeding positions for infants at the breast.
13. Counsel mothers who want to use or who are prescribed medications while they are breastfeeding.
14. Become adept at teaching mothers the use of alternative feeding methods.
15. Develop adeptness at working with mothers and infants with a variety of conditions that impact breastfeeding.
16. Acquire breastfeeding consultancy hours in preparation for sitting the IBLCE examination.

Evaluation Methods

Learning will be assessed by:

☐ Written didactics: condition specific sheets from the workbook "Clinical Experience in Lactation: A Blueprint for Internship, 2nd edition" 2010 (available from ILCA.org). At least 75 % will be completed satisfactorily prior to clinical hours being scheduled.

☐ Observation of clinical practice of the participant

☐ Pre-clinical and post-clinical conferences with an experienced IBCLC mentor

☐ Written patient experience summaries (reviewed by mentor, with satisfactory rating)

Feedback is given verbally as well as in written form. Written feedback uses daily evaluation forms during the first 50 clinical hours, then weekly/monthly evaluation forms, as negotiated by mentor and intern (based on the frequency and schedule of clinical days).

Clinical Environment

All units where lactation visits occur at CMC-NorthEast will be incorporated in the internship. Additional sites (e.g. health department, physician offices, other clinical care sites) may be contracted for completion of needed/desired clinical experiences.

Required Textbooks

"Clinical Experience In Lactation: A Blueprint for Internship, 2nd edition" by Barger and Kutner, available from ILCA.org or from the authors at Lactation Education Resources lactationeducationresources.com).

At least one comprehensive lactation management textbook (see resource list at IBLCE.org), such as Lawrence, Riordan, or Lauwers.

Computer access and skill in locating resources from medical and allied health professional literature (Assistance/guidance with learning this process can be arranged through AHEC, or the medical library on site at CMC-NorthEast).

Access to a number of the other resources listed in the resource list at IBLCE.org (Hale, core curriculum, etc.). Some of these will be available for on-site use at the Lactation Service office at CMC_NorthEast.

Attendance Requirements

Participants are expected to attend all scheduled conferences, clinical hours, and scheduled meetings. Evidence of preparation for the learning activity is expected. Punctuality is essential. Unplanned, extensive, or repeated absences may result in failure to meet course objectives, or dismissal from the internship. See policies regarding evaluations and withdrawal/dismissal in the Participant Handbook.

Absences do not relieve interns of the responsibility for course content. Interns are responsible for planning make-up work with the Chief Mentor who considers individual intern's progress in meeting the course objectives, type of experience missed, availability of mentors, demands of the schedule and reason for absence. A physician's verification for illness may be required at the Chief Mentor's discretion (also see Health Policy in Participant Handbook).

Withdrawal

Review the withdrawal policies, and keep the Chief Mentor advised in cases of changes in circumstance.

E-mail Correspondence/Voice Mail

E-mail and voice mail are valuable communication tools for issues related to information and notifications. Notifications are needed for schedule changes, making appointments, and specific assignments. Mentors will supply participants with their e-mail address. Voice mail messages may be left via the Lactation Service phone 704-403-1186.

In general, where there is a need to resolve differences regarding performance evaluation or academic issues, communication will be through a scheduled face-to-face meeting between the intern and mentor.

Academic Honesty Statement

Each lactation intern is expected to present herself in a manner of utmost integrity at all times, with all assignments. Collaboration and group study are encouraged in all learning activities. However, for individual written assignments, the intern must not collaborate with anyone in a manner that results in work that is not completely reflective of the individual intern's work. Cheating in any manner, which includes lying, stealing, unauthorized copying, falsification of records, or any dishonest act will result in disciplinary action. In particular, respect for copyrighted materials, with appropriate quotation, attribution, and citations are mandatory. The lactation intern is expected to abide by the Lactation Consultant Code of Ethics (see IBLCE.org).

Intern Identification

Lactation interns are required to wear ID badges at all times while in a clinical setting, worn above the waist, with picture and name visible at all times. The intern is to introduce herself appropriately, clearly defining her role as necessary, to all patients and colleagues.

General Information about Written Assignments

All assignments that have more than one page need to be turned in either stapled or in some form of folder or notebook, with the intern's name on each page. Assignments may be e-mailed to the mentor. Hand written assignments will be accepted only if the handwriting is clear and legible.

Course Outline

Note: Some of the Preliminary Steps Occur Prior to Clinical Hours

1. Complete comprehensive lactation management course
2. Submit application with fee
3. Complete Application Checklist
4. Interview
5. Acceptance decision/notification
6. Pay tuition deposit
7. Completion of enrollment checklist (health screening, ACE, CPR, insurance)

8. Chief Mentor will assist with scheduling orientation
9. Acquire required texts, including the required workbook "Clinical Experience in Lactation: A Blueprint for Internship, 2nd edition" and other lactation texts (see recommended resources at IBLCE.org).
10. As soon as accepted to the internship program, during completion of enrollment checklist, intern should begin completing didactic sheets on maternal and infant conditions from the workbook.
11. Receive periodic feedback on didactic sheets.
12. Submit internship approval forms to IBLCE (see IBLCE.org Pathway 3 Guide for forms and deadlines). Chief Mentor will supply program information.
13. When 75% of didactics completed successfully, and orientation complete, arrange schedule with Chief Mentor for clinical hours to begin
14. Tuition payment due at first clinical hours
15. Complete self evaluation of current knowledge/skills on competency skills checklist
16. Begin observation hours
17. Receive daily evaluations first approximately 50 hours/7 days, then weekly/monthly depending on schedule
18. Daily pre and post conferences with Chief Mentor or assigned Mentor
19. Complete individual patient write-up and clinical log daily (maintaining HIPAA at all times)
20. Receive feedback on written work at least weekly
21. Periodically review progress (review skills self-evaluation), logs, completion records, and revise schedule as needed with Mentors
22. Pay remaining tuition according to designated schedule
23. Completion of all competency checklist skills, and at least 90% of contacted activities from the workbook, increasing independent clinical care under supervision of mentor(s).
24. Final evaluation of participant, and evaluations by participant (of mentors and of program)
25. Completion checklist
26. Completion certificate awarded
27. Verification sent to IBLCE
28. Apply for IBLCE exam (mentor available to assist as needed)

Adapted from PTA Fieldwork syllabi

6/17/2010, 8/10/2010

Used with Permission Cabarrus College of Health Sciences, Concord, NC

Appendix 4

Checklists And Worksheets

CLINICAL COMPETENCIES CHECKLIST

CLINICAL EXPERIENCE LOG

ENGORGEMENT WORKSHEET

HYPERBILIRUBINEMIA WORKSHEET

COMPETENCIES FOR LACTATION CONSULTANT INTERNS

These competencies were printed by Lactation Education Consultants (LEC) in their 3rd edition of *Clinical Experience in Lact for Internship* and were adapted from the International Board of Lactation Consultant Examiners, April 2010 from IBLCE's G *a Mentored Lactation Education Plan: Pathway 3*. Notations that are in italics are LEC's expansion of IBCLE's competencies t the competency into their important and essential components. Some of the competencies are listed in a different order fr by IBLCE. This was done in an attempt to make it easier for the lactation intern to follow. Activities in this document that fo IBLCE competency are highlighted in bold.

Source: Kutner, LA, Barger, J. *Clinical Experience in Lactation: A Blueprint for Internship. 3rd edition.* 2010. Lactation Educatic Wheaton, Illinois, USA. © 2010 Lactation Education Consultants – Used with permission.

Communication and Counseling Skills

A. In all interactions with mothers, families, health care professionals and peers, the student will demonstrate effective cc to maintain collaborative and supportive relationships.

The student will:

	Competency	Competency Achieved	Comments
1	Identify factors that might affect communications (i.e., culture/language differences, deafness, vision problems, mental ability, etc)		
2	Demonstrate appropriate body language (i.e., position in relations to the other persons, comfortable eye contact, appropriate tone of voice for the setting, etc.)		
3	Demonstrate knowledge of and sensitivity to cultural differences		
A	*Incorporate such findings into the dyad's plan of care*		
4	Elicit information using effective counseling techniques (i.e., asking open-ended questions, summarizing the discussion, and providing emotional support).		
5	Make appropriate referrals to other health care professionals and community resources		

B. The student will provide individualized breastfeeding care with an emphasis on the mother's ability to make informed

The student will:

	Competency	Competency Achieved	Comments
6	Assess mother's psychological state and provide information appropriate to her situation.		
7	Include in discussion those family members or friends the mother identifies as significant to her.		
8	Obtain the mother's permission for hands-on assessment of her and the baby		
A	*Written forms*		
B	*Verbal permission*		
9	Ascertain mother's knowledge about and goals for breastfeeding.		
10	Use adult education principles to provide instruction to the mother that will meet her needs.		
11	Select appropriate written information and other teaching aids.		
A	*Materials adhere to the International Code of Marketing of Breastmilk Substitute guidelines*		
B	*Materials are at an appropriate literacy level.*		
C	*Materials do not contain pictures of breastfeeding equipment that the mother may not need.*		

History Taking and Assessment Skills

The student will be able to:

		Competency	Competency Achieved	Comments
1		Obtain a pertinent history		
	A	*Identifies which questions are important to ask in the inpatient setting based on the pregnancy, labor and delivery, and the condition of the dyad*		
	B	*Identifies which questions are important to ask in the outpatient setting based on the presenting complaint, ages of dyad, assessments and evaluations.*		
2		Perform a breast evaluation related to lactation		
	A	*Identifies both normal and abnormal findings*		
	B	*Identifies how findings are or may impact lactation*		
	C	*Documents findings appropriately*		
3		Develop a breastfeeding risk assessment		
	A	*Identifies physical findings which may have a negative impact on breastfeeding*		
	B	*Identifies facts from the history which may have a negative impact on breastfeeding*		
4		Assess and evaluates the infant relative to his ability to breastfeed.		
	A	*Able to identify physical findings that can have either a positive or negative impact on breastfeeding*		
	B	*Able to identify influences that can have either a positive or negative impact on the infant's ability to breastfeeding*		
5		Assess effective milk transfer		
	A	*Observes the infant for proper latch-on and for satiation cues*		
	B	*Questions infant's output and growth patterns*		
	C	*Assesses milk transfer using before and after feeding (AC/PC) weights*		
	D	*Observes mother for comfort with the feeding, and signs of prolactin and oxytocin release*		

Documentation and Communication Skills with Health Care Professionals

The student will:

	Competency	Competency Achieved	Comments
1	Communicate effectively with other members of the health care team, using appropriate written documents appropriate to the geopolitical region, facility and culture in which the student is being trained such as: 1.1 Consent forms 1.2 Charting forms/clinical notes 1.3 Pathways/care maps 1.4 Feeding assessment forms		
2	Use appropriate resources for research to provide information to the health care team on conditions, modalities and medications that affect breastfeeding and lactation		
3	Write referral and follow-up documentation/letters to referring and/or primary health care providers that illustrate the student's ability to identify: 3.1. The mother's concerns or problems, planned interventions, evaluation of outcomes and follow-up 3.2 Situations in which immediate verbal communication with the health care provider is necessary, such as serious illness in the infant, child, or the mother		
4	Report instances of child abuse or neglect to specific agencies as mandated or appropriate		

Skills for the First Two Hours After Birth

The student will:

	Competency	Competency Achieved	Comments
1	Identify events that occurred during the labor and birth process that may negatively impact breastfeeding.		
2	Identify and discourage practices (that occurred during labor and delivery) that may interfere with breastfeeding		
3	Promote continuous skin to skin contact of the term newborn and mother through the first feeding		
4	Assist mother and family to identify feeding cues		
5	Help mother and infant to find comfortable positions for attachment during the initial feeding after birth		
6	Identify correct latch-on (attachment)		
7	Reinforce to mother and family the importance of:		
	7.1 Keeping mother and infant together		
	7.2 Feeding baby on cue, but at least 8 times in 24 hours		

Postpartum Skills

Prior to discharge from care, the student will observe feedings and effectively instruct mothers about:

		Competency	Competency Achieved	Comments
1		Assessment of adequate milk intake by the baby		
	A	Correct latch (attachment)		
	B	Assessment of mother's comfort with the latch (attachment)		
	C	Assessment of the infant's output and weight patterns		
2		Normal infant sucking patterns		
	A	During a feed		
	B	During the first 24 hours		
	C	After the first 24 hours of life		
3.		How milk is produced, supply maintained, including discussion of growth/appetite spurts		
	A	Able to explain to the mother and family how milk is produced, maintained and increased		
	B	Able to explain to the mother and family what a growth spurt is, how to identify it, and how to deal with it		
4		Normal newborn behavior, including why, when and how to wake a sleepy baby		
5		Avoidance of early pacifier use and bottle nipples		
6		Importance of exclusive breastmilk feeds and possible consequences of mixed feedings with cow milk or soy		
7		Prevention and treatment of sore nipples		
8		Prevention and treatment of engorgement		
9		SIDS prevention behaviors		
10		Family planning methods and their relationships to breastfeeding		

		Competency	Competency Achieved	Comments
11		Education regarding drugs (such as nicotine, alcohol, caffeine and illicit drugs) and folk remedies (such as herbal teas)		
	A	Use of appropriate medical reference and referrals		
12		Plans for follow-up care for breastfeeding questions, infant's medical and mother's postpartum examinations		
13		Community resources for assistance with breastfeeding.		

Problem Solving Skills

The student will be able to:

	Competency	Competency Achieved	Comments
1	Identify problems *(that impact or may impact breastfeeding)*		
2	Assess contributing factors and etiology		
3	Develop an appropriate breastfeeding plan of care in concert with the mother		
4	Assist the mother to implement the plan		
5	Evaluate effectiveness of plans of care		

Skills for Maternal Breastfeeding Challenges

The student will be able to assist mothers with the following challenges:

		Competency	Competency Achieved	Comments
1		Cesarean Birth		
	A	*Assists mother with positions that are comfortable for nursing*		
	B	*Identifies impact of postpartum pain medications on the mother and infant*		
2		Flat or inverted nipples		
	A	*Assists mother with positioning of the infant and her hands to maximize the infant's ability to grasp the nipple*		
	B	*Recommends and assists the mother with devices to make it easier for the infant to grasp the nipple*		
3		Yeast *(and bacterial)* infections of the breast, nipple, areola and milk ducts		
	A	*Identify probable cause from history*		
	B	*Assessment of maternal milk supply*		
	C	*Assessment of infant for yeast infection*		
	D	*Appropriate referrals as needed*		
	E	*Knowledge of and appropriate use of antifungal, antibacterial and anti-inflammatory modalities*		
	F	*Develop appropriate plan of care*		
	G	*Evaluate effectiveness of plan of care*		
	H	*Change plan of care if necessary*		
4		Nipple pain and damage		
	A	*Identifies etiology*		

		Competency	Competency Achieved	Comments
	B	Assessment of maternal milk supply		
	C	Knowledge of and appropriate use of modalities used in the treatment of sore nipples		
	D	Develops appropriate plan of care		
	E	Evaluates outcome and changes plan of care as needed		
5		Engorgement		
	A	Identifies etiology		
	B	Develops appropriate plan of care using acceptable modalities such as heat/cold, use of cabbage, milk expression, etc.		
	C	Evaluates outcome and changes plan of care as needed		
6		Plugged Duct		
	A	Identifies etiology		
	B	Develops appropriate plan of care		
	C	Evaluates outcome within appropriate time frame		
7		Plugged Nipple Pore		
	A	Identifies etiology		
	B	Develops appropriate plan of care		
	C	Evaluates outcome and changes plan of care as needed		
8		Mastitis		
	A	Identifies etiology		
	B	Develops appropriate plan of care		
	C	Makes appropriate referrals as needed		
	D	Evaluates outcome in a timely manner and changes plan of care as needed		
9		Insufficient milk supply, differentiating between perceived and real		
	A	Identifies etiology		
	B	Differentiates between perceived and real insufficient milk supply		
	C	Using AC/PC weights and Milk Intake Sheet to assess supply and infant's ability to transfer milk		
	D	Develops appropriate care plan		
	E	Evaluates outcome in a timely manner and makes changes in plan of care as needed		
10		Breast surgery or trauma		
	A	Identifies and is able to describe the various types of breast surgery and how they can impact breastfeeding		
	B	Asks questions regarding possible breast trauma and is able to relate how this can impact breastfeeding		
	C	Evaluates milk supply when a history of breast surgery or trauma is given		
	D	Develops an appropriate plan of care		
	E	Evaluates outcome in a timely manner and changes plan of care as needed		
11		Overproduction of milk		

		Competency	Competency Achieved	Comments
	A	*Identifies problems that occur in mother and infant with overproduction*		
	B	*Knowledge of and appropriate use of means to reduce milk supply*		
	C	*Does feeding assessment to differentiate between this condition and others with similar symptoms*		
	D	*Develops appropriate plan of care*		
	E	*Evaluates outcome in a timely manner and changes plan of care as needed*		
12		Cultural beliefs that are not evidence based and may interfere with breastfeeding, (i.e., discarding colostrum, rigidly scheduling feedings, necessity of a breastmilk substitute after every breastfeeding, etc.)		
	A	*Works appropriately with the mother, family and staff to enhance breastfeeding while taking cultural beliefs into consideration*		
13		Medical conditions that impact breastfeeding		
	A	*Identifies medical conditions and is able to identify the risk it may present to breastfeeding and to develop appropriate plans of care*		
	B	*Diabetes*		
	C	*Pregnancy Induced Hypertension*		
	D	*Eclampsia*		
	E	*Excessive blood loss*		
	F	*Infertility problems*		
14		Adolescent mother		
		14.1 Strategies for returning to school		
		14.1 Strategies for returning to school		
		14.2 Maintaining milk supply		
15		Continuation of breastfeeding when mother is separated from her baby		
		15.1 Milk expression technique		
		15.2 Maintaining milk production		
		15.3 Collection, storage and transportation of milk		
	A	*Supporting mother who is separated from her infant*		
16		Postpartum psychological issues including transient sadness ('baby blues'), and postpartum depression		
		16.1 Appropriate referrals		
		16.2 Medications compatible with breastfeeding		
17		Weaning issues		
		17.1 Safe formula preparation and feeding techniques		
		17.2 Care of breasts		

Skills for Infant Breastfeeding Challenges

The student will be able to assist mothers who have infants with the following challenges:

		Competency	Competency Achieved	Comments
1		Traumatic birth		
	A	*Identification of factors leading to diagnosis of traumatic birth*		
	B	*Identification and management of risk factors influenced by lactation*		
	C	*Development of appropriate feeding plan*		
2		35-38 weeks gestation		
		34-38 weeks of completed gestation ... late preterm infant		
	A	*Identification of risk factors associated with the late preterm infant*		
	B	*Identification and management of risk factors influenced by lactation*		
	C	*Insurance pumping*		
	D	*Development of appropriate feeding plan*		
	E	*Timely follow-up*		
3		Small for gestational age (SGA)		
	A	*Identification of risk factors associated with SGA infants*		
	B	*Identification and management of risk factors influenced by lactation*		
4		Large for gestational age (LGA)		
	A	*Identification of risk factors associated with LGA infants*		
	B	*Identification and management of risk factors influenced by lactation*		
	C	*Development of appropriate feeding plan*		
	D	*Insurance pumping*		
	E	*Timely follow-up*		
5		Multiples/plural births		
	A	*Identification of risk factors associated with plural births*		
	B	*Identification and management of risk factors influenced by lactation*		
	C	*Positioning for simultaneous nursing*		
	D	*Development of appropriate feeding plan*		
	E	*Recommendations for dealing with required activities of daily living*		
6		Preterm birth, including the benefits of kangaroo care		
	A	*Identification of risk factors associated with preterm infants*		
	B	*Identification and management of risk factors influenced by lactation*		
	C	*Lactoengineering/fractionating when appropriate*		
	D	*Maintaining milk supply while infant is in the hospital*		
	E	*Maintaining supply after the infant is discharged*		
	F	*Knowledge of and with assisting with kangaroo care*		

		Competency	Competency Achieved	Comments
	G	*Knowledge of and assisting with appropriate supplemental feeding methods*		
	H	*Recommendations for dealing with required activities of daily living*		
	I	*Development of appropriate feeding plan*		
7		High risk for hypoglycemia		
	A	*Identification of risk factors*		
	B	*Identification and management of risk factors influenced by lactation*		
	C	*Knowledge of and assisting with appropriate feeding methods*		
	D	*Knowledge of and assisting with appropriate kinds of supplements*		
8		Sleepy (difficult to rouse)		
	A	*Identification and management of risk factors that can be influenced by lactation*		
	B	*Use of appropriate gentle waking practices*		
	C	*Development of appropriate feeding plan*		
9		Excessive weight loss (failure to thrive)		
	A	*Identification of possible maternal causes*		
	B	*Identification of possible maternal causes*		
	C	*Assessment of maternal milk production*		
	D	*Assessment of infant's ability to transfer milk*		
	E	*Ability to calculate need for supplementation*		
	F	*Knowledge of and assisting with appropriate alternative feeding methods*		
	G	*Knowledge of and assisting with appropriate kinds of supplementation*		
	H	*Milk expression to increase supply*		
	I	*Appropriate use of galactagogues*		
	J	*Development of appropriate feeding plan*		
	K	*Timely follow-up*		
10		Slow or poor weight gain		
	A	*Differentiation between slow weight gain and poor weight gain*		
	B	*Identification of possible maternal causes*		
	C	*Identification of possible infant causes*		
	D	*Review of growth patterns of parents and other children in the family*		
	E	*Assessment of maternal milk production*		
	F	*Assessment of infant's ability to transfer milk*		
	G	*Ability to calculate amount of supplementation if needed*		
	H	*Appropriate feeding plan*		
	I	*Timely follow up*		
11		Hyperbilirubinemia (jaundice)		
	A	*Identifies risk factors associated with hyperbilirubinemia*		

		Competency	Competency Achieved	Comments
	B	Identification and management of risk factors that can be influenced by lactation		
	C	Identifies different types of hyperbilirubinemia and effect lactation has on each		
	D	Appropriate feeding plan		
12		Ankyloglossia (short frenulum)		
	A	Identifies risk factors associated with ankyloglossia for both mother and infant		
	B	Evaluates mobility of the infant's tongue		
	C	Assesses infant's ability to transfer milk		
	D	Assesses mother's milk supply		
	E	Assesses infant's growth		
	F	Makes appropriate referrals as needed		
	G	Arranges timely follow up		
13		Yeast infection (thrush)		
	A	Identification risk factors in both mother and infant		
	B	Appropriate referrals if needed		
	C	Appropriate plan of care in regards to environment, feeds, and infected area(s)		
14		Colic/fussiness		
	A	Identification of possible risk factors in both mother and infant		
	B	Addressing the elimination of possible causes		
	C	Development of appropriate plan of care		
	D	Techniques and/or modalities for making the infant more comfortable		
	E	Emotional support for parents		
	F	Teaching normal newborn behaviors		
	G	Appropriate follow up		
15		Gastric reflux		
	A	Identification of possible risk factors		
	B	Identification of possible causes (i.e. cow's milk protein)		
	C	Identification of possible complications (i.e. poor weight gain, aspiration, oral aversion)		
	D	Assessment of mother's milk supply		
	E	Assessment of infant's milk intake		
	F	Techniques and/or modalities for making the infant more comfortable		
	G	Appropriate feeding plan		
	H	Timely follow up		
16		Lactose overload (low fat feeds, hyperlactation syndrome, breastmilk imbalance)		
	A	Identification of possible causes		
	B	Identification of possible complications		
	C	Assessment of mother's milk supply		

		Competency	Competency Achieved	Comments
	D	Assessment of infant's milk intake		
	E	Methods to decrease mother's milk supply		
	F	Techniques and/or modalities for making the infant more comfortable		
	G	Appropriate plan of care		
	H	Timely follow up		
17		Food intolerance		
	A	Identification of possible causes		
	B	Analyzing mother's food diary		
	C	Identification of possible complications		
	D	Development of appropriate maternal diet		
	E	Maternal nutritional support as needed		
	F	Appropriate plan of care		
	G	Timely follow up		
18		Neurodevelopmental problems		
	A	Identification of problems that can effect lactation		
	B	Appropriate feeding plan		
	C	Timely follow up		
19		Teething and biting		
	A	Identification of possible causes		
	B	Appropriate suggestions to mother		
20		Nursing strikes/early baby-led weaning		
	A	Identification of possible causes		
	B	Appropriate suggestions to mother		
	C	Maintaining milk supply		
21		Toddler nursing		
	A	Identification of possible problems		
	B	Appropriate suggestions to mother		
22		Nursing through pregnancy		
	A	Identification of possible problems		
	B	Appropriate suggestions to mother		
23		Tandem nursing		
	A	Identification of possible problems		
	B	Appropriate feeding patterns for both the newborn and older child		
	C	Nursing positions for simultaneous nursing		
	D	Appropriate suggestions to the mother		
	E	Assistance and advice for weaning the toddler if mother decides to wean		

Management Skills

The student will demonstrate the ability to:

	Competency	Competency Achieved	Comments
1	Perform a comprehensive breastfeeding assessment		
2	Assess milk transfer with:		
	2.1 AC/PC weights, using an electronic digital scale		
3	Calculate an infant's caloric and volume requirements		
4	Use a balance (beam) scale for daily weights		
5	Increase mother's milk production		
A	*Plans for more effective nursing*		
B	*Appropriate use of galactagogues*		
C	*Plans for additional milk expression*		

Skills For Use Of Technology And Devices

The student will have up-to-date knowledge about breastfeeding-related equipment and demonstrate appropriate use and understanding of potential disadvantages or risks of the following:

	Competency	Competency Achieved	Comments
1	A device to evert nipples		
2	Nipple creams/ointments		
3	Breast shells		
4	Breast pumps		
5	Alternative feeding techniques		
	5.1 Tube feeding at the breast		
	5.2 Cup feeding		
	5.3 Spoon feeding		
	5.4 Eyedropper feeding		
	5.5 Finger feeding		
	5.6 Bottle and artificial nipples		
6	Nipple shields		
7	Pacifiers		
8	Infant scales		
9	Use of herbal supplements for mother and/or infant		

Skills for Breastfeeding Challenges Encountered Infrequently

The following issues are encountered relatively infrequently, and may not be seen during the student's training. The entry-level lactation consultant would not be expected to be proficient in these situations. The student will need to use basic skills to assist the mother and infant while seeking guidance from a more experienced IBCLC

A. Infant Issues

	IBLCE Stated Competency	Competency Achieved	Comments
1	Infant with tonic bite/ineffective/dysfunctional suck		
2	Cranial-facial abnormalities		
	2.1 Micrognathia (receding lower jaw)		
	2.2 Cleft lip and/or palate		
3	Down Syndrome		
4	Cardiac problems		
5	Chronic medical problems such as cystic fibrosis, PKU, etc.		

B.   Maternal Issues

	Stated Competency	Competency Achieved	Comments
1	Induced lactation		
2	Relactation		
3	Coping with the death of an infant		
4	Chronic medical conditions, such as: 4.1 MS 4.2 Lupus 4.3 Seizures 4.4 Others		
5	Disabilities which may limit mother's ability to handle the baby easily, such as rheumatoid arthritis, carpal tunnel syndrome, cerebral palsy, etc.		
6	HIV/AIDS: understanding of current recommendations based on the mother's access to safe replacement feeding		

Skills for Meeting Professional Responsibility

The student will demonstrate the following professional responsibilities:

	Competency	Competency Achieved	Comments
1	Conduct herself or himself in a professional manner, by complying with the IBLCE Code of Professional Conduct for International Board Certified Lactation Consultants and the ILCA Standards of Practice; and by adhering to the International Code of the Marketing of Breast-Milk Substitutes and its subsequent World Health Assembly Resolutions		
2	Practice within the laws of the setting in which s/he works, showing respect for confidentiality and privacy		
3	Utilize current research findings to provide a strong evidence base for clinical practice, and obtain continuing education to enhance skills and obtain/maintain IBCLC certification		
4	Advocate for breastfeeding families, mothers, infants and children in the workplace, community and within the health care system		
5	Use breastfeeding equipment appropriately and provide information about risks as well as benefits of products, maintaining an awareness of conflict of interest if profiting from the rental or sale of breastfeeding equipment		

Sites The Student May Use For Acquisition Of Skills

It is most helpful if the student utilizes as many of the following sites for acquisition of skills as possible:

	Competency	Competency Achieved	Comments
1	Private practice IBCLC office		
2	Private practice OB, pediatric, family practice or midwifery office		
3	Public Health Department; Women, Infants and Children (WIC) Program (in the U.S.)		
4	Hospital		
	4.1 Lactation services		
	4.2 Birthing center (Labor and Delivery		

	Competency	Competency Achieved	Comments
	4.3 Postpartum Unit		
	4.4 Mother/Baby Unit		
	4.5 Level II and Level III nurseries: Special Care Nursery, Neonatal Intensive Care Unit		
	4.6 Pediatric Unit		
5	Home health services		
6	Outpatient follow-up breastfeeding clinics		
7	Breastfeeding hotlines & warmlines		
8	Prenatal and postpartum breastfeeding classes		
9	Volunteer community support group meetings		
10	Home births (if legally permitted)		

LOG FOR CLINICAL PRACTICE HOURS

DATE	SITE	EXPERIENCE	TIME	MENTOR(S)	Mentor Approval
(Example) 5/7/2013	Hospital	Baby A: reluctant nurser, position and latch Mother B: pumping instructions Mother C: Hx PCOS very anxious Baby D: tongue tie, consult, nipple shield, supp	3 hours	L. Kutner	LK

Mother with Engorged Breasts

1. Describe the different degrees of engorgement.

2. What factors contribute to the development of engorgement?

3. What women are more likely to develop engorgement?

4. What is the possible sequella for unrelieved engorgement?

5. What are the possible outcomes for both the mother and infant when a mother has +++ or ++++ engorgement?

6. What factors associated with the infant can contribute to this condition?

7. How was engorgement treated in the past? Why were these treatments frequently ineffective?

8. If icy compresses are recommended for engorgement, when should they be used? How long will you recommend they be used on the breast at one time?

9. If cabbage is recommended for this condition, how will you recommend it be used? What are the side effects of using cabbage?

10. What is Reverse Pressure Softening? How would you use it in this case?

11. Is it appropriate to recommend the mom use a breast pump for engorgement? If so, how would you suggest it be used?

12. What would be your recommendation for nursing while a mother is engorged?

13. What medications might a mother take when she is engorged? Explain how these medications work.

Source: Kutner, LA, Barger, J. Clinical Experience in Lactation: A Blueprint for Internship. 3rd edition. 2010. Lactation Education Consultants: Wheaton, Illinois, USA. Copyright © 2010 Lactation Education Consultants – used with permission.

Infant with Hyperbilirubinemia

1. Describe the different kinds of jaundice that are seen in newborns?
2. What are the two types of jaundice that you are most likely to see in newborns?
3. How does bilirubin develop in a newborn?
4. List the conditions that can increase bilirubin in a newborn.
5. What is the danger of hyperbilirubinemia in a newborn?
    a. What levels are considered dangerous?
    b. How does the baby's age impact the danger level?
6. What are the current recommendations for treating jaundice?
7. What impact does giving the infant glucose water have on bilirubin levels?
8. What is the effect of frequent stooling on bilirubin levels?
9. What ethnic groups normally see higher bilirubin levels in their infants?
10. Is there anything good about elevated bilirubin levels in newborns?
11. What maternal factors can contribute to this condition?
12. What infant factors can contribute to this condition?
13. What suggestions could you make to a mother so that she could decrease the chance of her infant developing jaundice?
14. What are some of the responses parents have when their child is diagnosed with jaundice?
15. What is a frequent long-term parental response to this diagnosis?

Appendix 5

Evaluation Documents

Evaluation Process
Daily Evaluation Of Intern
Monthly Evaluation Of Intern
Final Evaluation Of Intern
Intern Self-Evaluation
Intern Evaluation Of Instructor
Intern Evaluation Of Program

LACTATION CLINICAL INTERNSHIP EVALUATIONS

Clinical Evaluation

Lactation Clinical Interns are evaluated in the clinical area using clinical outcomes and behaviors listed on the Intern Daily and Monthly Evaluation forms. The outcomes are based on the course objectives, and are designed to meet requirements for the IBCLE certification pathways. Interns are expected to achieve "satisfactory" ratings on all the clinical outcomes listed in the written evaluations. Interns will be evaluated on performance in various clinical areas related to lactation care, by the mentor assigned to them for the day.

For the first 7 clinical days (approximately 50 hours), the intern will be evaluated on each behavior listed on the Intern Daily Evaluation Form using the following scale:
- **5=Excellent**
- **4=Very Good**
- **3=Satisfactory**
- **2=Needs Improvement**
- **1=Unsatisfactory**

- Ongoing evaluations will occur monthly (or more often if arranged between the student and Chief Mentor), and will include ratings on the Lactation Clinical Internship Monthly Evaluation Form using the same scale.
- Two or more ratings of **2 or less** in an individual behavior indicate the intern is not meeting expectations.
- If an intern receives a rating of **2 or less** on any individual behavior for two consecutive evaluations, written remediation will be set up immediately by the interns and the mentor. **It is the intern's responsibility to discuss with/inform the Chief Mentor of this situation so it can be addressed immediately.** Failure to do so will result in a rating of "**not meeting expectations.**"
- **In addition to individual behavior evaluation, the intern will receive a rating of "did not meet expectations" overall for the following additional behaviors:**

  o **Unsafe Acts**
  o **Repeated Clinical Errors**
  o **Violating Confidentiality**
  o **Being Unprepared for Clinical**
  o **Failure to Demonstrate Progression in Clinical Performance**
  o **Unprofessional Behaviors**
  o **Failure to complete written assignments and/or failure to turn in on time**
  o **Repeated occurrences of the above behaviors after remediation will result in being unsatisfactory in clinical**
  o **No call, no show, repeated tardiness**

7/20/2010

- **Two "did not meet expectations" clinical evaluations without effective remediation will result in an unsatisfactory rating in the course, and may result in dismissal.**
- **If the intern is asked to leave the clinical area due to professional or personal conflicts that cannot be resolved, the intern will be asked to leave the internship program and receive an unsatisfactory clinical evaluation.**
- A conference will be held if necessary and scheduled by the intern. The student will not be allowed to continue in clinical until arrangements have been made for a meeting. Interns will be counseled on any rating of **Needs Improvement.**
- Attending clinical as scheduled is essential in meeting the expected outcomes.
    1. For clinical absences, notify the lactation office (704-403-1186) no later than 0700 the day of the absence.
    2. All clinical hours will require completion of makeup time.
    3. More than 10% unplanned absences will result in failure to meet the objective of the course and result in unsatisfactory clinical evaluation.
    4. An episode of "no call, no show" for clinical practicum will be addressed as follows:
        a) First episode will include verbal counseling of the intern with a written memo to the intern's record.
        b) Second episode may result in the intern being dismissed from the Clinical Lactation Internship program.

Intern responsibilities will include:
- Interns will participate in facility and departmental orientation.
- A clinical work schedule will be collaboratively established with the mentor(s). The mentor(s) must approve all changes.
- Interns are expected to arrive fifteen minutes before the start of the clinical experience.
- All written assignments will be turned in to the Chief Mentor for grading.
- A final evaluation will be done by the Chief Mentor.

Used with Permission Cabarrus College of Health Sciences, Concord, NC

7/20/2010

Carolinas Medical Center
NorthEast
Lactation Clinical Internship
DAILY EVALUATION

Intern's Name: _____ Date: _____

Work Site: _____
Clinical Experience(s):

Written Work _____ Completed _____ Incomplete (explain)

Evaluate on a scale of 1 to 5 [1 = Unsatisfactory 5 = Excellent]

History Taking	1	2	3	4	5
Maternal Assessment	1	2	3	4	5
Infant Assessment	1	2	3	4	5
Feeding Assessment	1	2	3	4	5
Plan of Care	1	2	3	4	5
Documentation	1	2	3	4	5
Follow-up	1	2	3	4	5
Counseling Skills	1	2	3	4	5
Professionalism	1	2	3	4	5

Strengths:

Weaknesses:

General comments:

_____   _____
Mentor's Signature/date   Intern's Signature/Date
Lactation Clinical Internship Participant Handbook
Adapted from BSC

Used with Permission Cabarrus College of Health Sciences, Concord, NC   7/20/10

INTERN MONTHLY EVALUATION

Intern's Name: _____   Month/Year_____

Experiences Encountered or Completed:						
Evaluate: [1=Needs improvement 5=Excellent]						**Comments**
History Taking	1	2	3	4	5	
Maternal Assessments	1	2	3	4	5	
Infant Assessments	1	2	3	4	5	
Feeding Assessments	1	2	3	4	5	
Plans of Care	1	2	3	4	5	
Charting	1	2	3	4	5	
Follow-up	1	2	3	4	5	
Counseling Skills	1	2	3	4	5	
Professionalism	1	2	3	4	5	
Strengths						
Weaknesses						
Suggestions for Improvement						

Comments:

_____   _____
Clinical Instructor's Signature   Intern's Signature

Carolinas Medical Center
NorthEast
Lactation Clinical Internship
FINAL EVALUATION

Intern's Name: _____ Date: _____

Primary clinical site_____

Primary Clinical Mentor_____ Contact_____ _____

Dates of Internship from _____ to _____

Description of Course/Program:

Evaluate on a scale of 1 to 5 [1 = Unsatisfactory 5 = Excellent]

Comment on strengths and weaknesses in each category:

History Taking	1	2	3	4	5
Maternal Assessments	1	2	3	4	5
Infant Assessments	1	2	3	4	5
Feeding Assessments	1	2	3	4	5
Plans of Care	1	2	3	4	5
Documentation	1	2	3	4	5
Follow-up	1	2	3	4	5
Counseling Skills	1	2	3	4	5
Professionalism	1	2	3	4	5

Overall strengths for practicing as an IBCLC :

Overall weaknesses for practicing as an IBCLC :

Suggestions:

Lactation Clinical Internship FINAL EVALUATION (page 2)

Do you believe that this Intern is prepared to sit for the next scheduled IBLCE examination?

___ Yes, the intern is ready to sit for the examination

___ No, the intern is not ready to sit for the examination

If you do not believe the intern is prepared to sit for the examination:

1. Please explain why

2. Please give suggestions that will help prepare the student for the examination.

_____   _____
Chief Mentor's Signature/date   Intern's Signature/Date
Lactation Clinical Internship Participant Handbook
Adapted from BSC
7/20/2010

Used with Permission Cabarrus College of Health Sciences, Concord, NC

Intern Self Evaluation

Lactation Consultant Skills	Expertise Level			Describe Your Experience
	ADV	INTERM	BASIC	
1.0 Education and Advocacy				
1.2 Review nutritional recommendations for lactation, provide written guidelines if necessary, and refer to a nutritionist or supplementary food program if needed.				
1.5 Discuss the effects of medications, illegal drugs, chemicals and home remedies on lactation and infant health (make specific recommendations)				
1.6 Act as an advocate for breastfeeding in the community, work place and within the health care professions.				
1.7 Act as an advocate for the breastfeeding family in the pursuit of optimal health care.				
1.9 Develop the necessary understanding of cultural differences in the community as they relate to breastfeeding				
2.0 Clinical Management of Breastfeeding				
2.1 Consent				
2.1.1 Obtain informed content from mother after identification of need for lactation consultant services is made.				
2.1.2 Obtain mother's permission to conduct assessment				
2.2 History				
2.2.1 Systematically obtain and update history of the mother and infant relative to lactation and breastfeeding, including pregnancy, labor, delivery, previous breastfeeding experiences, current breastfeeding experiences including feeding, elimination and sleep patterns, and current health of mother and baby.				
2.2.2 Identify the possible conditions or problems based on history and assessment				
2.2.3 Evaluate the emotional status of the mother and the elements of her support system. Refer when indicated.				
2.3 Assessment/Examination				
2.3.1 Wash hands prior to examining mother or baby and maintain high standards of hygiene				
2.3.2 Examine the mother's breasts				
2.3.2.1 Nipple protractility and breast elasticity				
2.3.2.2 Lumps, breast obstructions, inflammation, edema, engorgement, scars, abnormal anatomy.				
2.3.2.3 Alterations breast & nipple skin integrity				
2.3.2.4 Breast, nipple and areola size, appearance and symmetry.				

Lactation Consultant Skills	Expertise Level ADV INTERM BASIC			Describe Your Experience
2.3.3 Examine and/or observe the infant during non-feeding times for:				
2.3.3.1 Level of alertness				
2.3.3.2 Level of irritability				
2.3.3.3 Body alignment and symmetry				
2.3.3.4 Muscle tone & activity, body & mouth				
2.3.3.5 Facial features and oral anatomy				
2.3.3.6 Weight, weight for length ratio; length, head, and chest circumference, and growth pattern since birth				
2.3.3.7 Hydration status				
2.3.3.8 Age appropriate reflexes and other developmental milestones				
2.3.4 Observe mother and infant during a feeding				
2.3.4.1 Observe body position of mother and baby				
2.3.4.2 Assess milk transfer				
2.3.4.3 Observe and assess milk intake, noting: Successful and proper attachment to breast, Breathing pattern at breast, Suckling pattern, Swallowing of milk				
2.4 Analysis				
2.4.1 Formulate and communicate a complete list of concerns, conditions, and/or problems and verify with the mother				
2.4.2 Provide information to enable the mother to make decisions & to assume responsibility for her own health & her infant's health and feeding plan				
2.4.3 Initiate crisis intervention management when indicated				
2.5 Recommendations				
2.5.1 Use accepted counseling techniques and communication skills with mothers and support persons				
2.5.2 Identify the need for consultation and referral to appropriate members of the health care team or community support resources.				
2.5.3 Develop with the mother a comprehensive feeding and care plan based on the history and assessment				
2.5.4 Evaluate with the mother possible goals and modify plans of care as needed.				
2.5.5 Provide written instructions to the mother				
2.6 Reporting and follow-up				
2.6.1 Keep accurate and complete records on findings and care provided for mother and baby				

Lactation Consultant Skills	Expertise Level			Describe Your Experience
	ADV	INTERM.	BASIC	
2.6.2 Regularly confer with and report progress, plans, and evaluations to all primary health workers caring for the mother and baby.				
2.6.3 Provide follow-up plans for each client contact.				
3.0 Technical Knowledge				
3.1 Demonstrate usual and special positioning techniques for mother and baby				
3.2 Select and explain assistance techniques based on history and assessment of the situation.				
3.2.1 Increase or decrease infant intake.				
3.2.3 Manual (hand) milk expression				
3.2.4 Safe and effective collection and storage of breastmilk				
3.2.5 Alternate massage				
3.2.6 Maternal diet modifications relative to sufficient intake, maternal or infant food intolerance, maternal or infant food allergies and their effect on the infant lactation.				
3.2.7 Finger-feeding with tubing, syringe, dropper				
3.3 Discuss the risk and benefits of the use of the following items:				
3.3.1 Breast pads				
3.3.2 Nipple creams and oils				
3.3.3 Nipple shields				
3.3.4 Nursing bras				
3.3.5 Slings and carries				
3.3.6 Nursing pillows				
3.3.7 Special clothing				
3.3.8 Pacifiers				
3.3.9 Mothers own milk, donors breastmilk and breastmilk substitutes.				
3.4 Select and explain equipment based on history and assessment of the situation.				
3.4.1 Breast pumps				
3.4.2 Breast shells				
3.4.3 Devices for dimpled nipples				
3.4.4 Alternative feeding devices				
3.4.4.1 feeding tube devices				
3.4.4.2 cups				
3.4.4.3 bottles with artificial nipples/teats				
3.4.4.4 droppers				
3.4.4.5 syringes				
3.4.4.6 spoons				
3.4.4.7 bowls				

4.0	Special Knowledge and assistance				
	Lactation Consultant Skills	**Expertise Level**			**Describe Your Experience**
		ADV	INTERM	BASIC	
4.1	Develop special plans for the continuation of breastfeeding if any of the following conditions are present in the infant. Assist the mother in implementing those plans.				
4.1.1	Hyperbilirubinemia				
4.1.2	Problems with attachment (latch-on)				
4.1.3	Dysfunctional, disorganized or weak suck				
4.1.4	"Nipple confusion" and nipple preference				
4.1.5	Breast preference				
4.1.6	Prematurity				
4.1.7	Postmaturity				
4.1.8	Temporary mother-baby separation				
4.1.9	Low birth weight				
4.1.10	Down Syndrome				
4.1.11	Developmental disability				
4.1.12	Physical challenges				
4.1.13	Neurological impairment				
4.1.14	Insufficient weight gain				
4.1.15	Cleft lip, cleft palate, and other orofacial abnormalities				
4.1.16	Digestive and metabolic disorders				
4.1.17	Infectious and contagious diseases				
4.1.18	Gastroenteritis				
4.1.19	Other illness/conditions that may adversely affect breastfeeding				
4.2	Develop special plans for the continuation of breastfeeding if any of the following conditions are present in the mother. Assist the mother in implementing those plans				
4.2.1	Breast engorgement				
4.2.2	Nipple problems and anomalies				
4.2.3	Breast pain				
4.2.4	Milk ejection problems				
4.2.5	Obstructed milk duct				
4.2.6	Infections and non-infectious mastitis				
4.2.7	Breast abscess				
4.2.8	Cystic breast disease				
4.2.9	Variations in milk supply				
4.2.10	Breast surgery				
4.2.11	Cesarean birth				
4.2.12	Induced lactation and relactation				
4.2.13	Endocrine disorders				
4.2.14	Enzyme deficiencies & metabolic disorders				
4.2.15	Seizure disorders				

Lactation Consultant Skills	Expertise Level			Describe Your Experience
	ADV	INTERM	BASIC	
4.2.17 Physical challenges				
4.2.18 Adolescence				
4.2.19 Infectious and contagious diseases				
4.2.20 Acute or chronic medication				
4.2.21 Recreational drug use				
4.2.22 Other illness/conditions that may adversely affect BF				
4.3 Develop and assist the mother in the implementation of special plans for the following situation:				
4.3.1 Separation from infant				
4.3.2 Working and Breastfeeding				
4.3.3 Relinquishing the infant for adoption				
4.3.4 Death of the infant				
5.0 Professional Responsibilities & Activities				
5.1 Identify the need for consultation and collaboration with other members of the health care team. Make referrals to:				
5.1.1 Peer or lay support groups				
5.1.2 Other IBCLC with specific expertise				
5.1.3 Physician, nurse practitioner, midwife, specialist, physical therapist, occupational therapist or other health care specialist				
5.2 Coordinate services with other health care workers				
5.2.1 Consult and confer with other lactation consultants as needed				
5.2.2 Inform client of consultations with other resources				
5.3 Make provisions for coverage outside of normal practice hours.				
5.4 Pursue continuing education relevant to lactation consultant practice, including reading current professional journals, participation in workshops, seminars, in-service programs, conferences, accredited courses.				
5.4.1 Present evidence of maintaining and expanding knowledge and skills through participation in any other professional development activities				
5.5 Support the development of relevant education and certification process for the lactation consultant profession				
5.6 Assess equipment safety and effectiveness				
5.7 Observe guidelines for health workers in the International Code of Marketing of Breastmilk Substitutes.				
5.8 Maintain professional credibility through membership in appropriate professional organizations				
5.9 Initiate, participate in, & report on research in the field of human lactation as opportunities arise				

Lactation Consultant Skills	Expertise Level ADV	INTERM	BASIC	Describe Your Experience
5.10 Act as a resource to peer support groups				
5.11 Create peer support groups as indicated				
5.12 Create & staff Breastfeeding hotline as needed				
5.13 Rent or sell breastfeeding equipment as desired				
5.14 When advertising the lactation consultant practice in any media, use the following guidelines, whether through telephone directory, periodicals, displays, newspapers, radio, television, written communications or other media:				
5.14.1 Reflect support of the International Code of Marketing of Breastmilk Substitutes in all advertising.				
5.14.2 Make no advertising claim which cannot be met in full without further qualifications; provide accurate information regarding services and products.				
5.14.3 Advertise in a manner which conforms to generally accepted standards of good taste; avoid practices, words and illustrations that may be offensive				
5.14.4 Retain a copy or recording of advertisement				
6.0 Business Practices/Legal Considerations				
6.1 Maintain patient confidentiality				
6.2 Charge reasonable fees for services rendered, as determined by local community norms for comparable health care				
6.3 Make a clear statement to the mother regarding fees and billing prior to providing services				
6.4 Obtain written release when photographing a mother and/or baby				
6.5 Carry appropriate malpractice insurance coverage				
6.6 Follow local laws and codes				
6.7 Maintain patient records for an appropriate time period.				

Comments:

Carolinas Medical Center
NorthEast

Lactation Clinical Internship
Intern's Evaluation of Clinical Mentor(s)

Name of mentor being evaluated:_____

1. Please rate your mentor's helpfulness in your mastery of the following areas:

Evaluate on a scale of 1 to 5 [1 = Unsatisfactory 5 = Excellent]

History Taking	1	2	3	4	5
Maternal Assessment	1	2	3	4	5
Infant Assessment	1	2	3	4	5
Feeding Assessment	1	2	3	4	5
Plan of Care	1	2	3	4	5
Charting	1	2	3	4	5
Follow-up	1	2	3	4	5
Counseling Skills	1	2	3	4	5
Professionalism	1	2	3	4	5

2. Please comment of the assistance and supervision you received from your mentor.

Describe ways in which your mentor was most helpful.

Describe ways in which your mentor could have been more helpful.

Additional Comments:

_____/_____ _____
Intern's Signature/Print Intern's name (optional)   Date

Please return completed form to Nurse Manager of Lactation Services.
Lactation Clinical Internship Participant Handbook
Adapted from BSC 7/20/10

Used with Permission Cabarrus College of Health Sciences, Concord, NC

Carolinas Medical Center
NorthEast

Lactation Clinical Internship
Intern's Evaluation of Program

Name: _____ Date: _____

_____
Street Address   City   State   Zip/Postal Code

Day Phone: _____   E-mail: _____

Primary Mentor: _____

Dates of Internship from: _____ to _____

1. Description of On-site Experience:

2. Description of Off-Site Experience:

3. What were your expectations for this program?

   To what extent did the program meet your expectations?

   Describe how this was accomplished.

4. Describe your overall "hands-on" experience at the on-site campus.

   How could this aspect of the program be improved?

   Which experiences seemed to be the most difficult to obtain?

   To what extent were you given adequate opportunities to do consultations by yourself?

5. To what extent did you find your off-site experiences helpful? Please explain.

   How easy or difficult did you find it to locate off-site experiences?

   Please describe your most helpful off-site experience.

   Please describe your least helpful off-site experience.

6. How helpful were the education conferences? Please explain.

   Describe those that were most helpful.

   Describe those that were least helpful.

   What additional education conferences would you suggest?

7. What do you think is the strength of this program?

8. What do you think is the weakness of this program?

9. What suggestions do you have for improving this program?

10. How helpful was this program in preparing you to take the ICLCE examination?

11. Do you feel you are ready to sit for the next offering of the IBLCE examination? If not, what additional preparation do you believe you need?

12. Do you feel that you have gained sufficient experience from this program to begin practice as a lactation consultant? If not, what additional experience do you believe you need?

Additional Comments:

_____
Intern's Signature/date (optional)

Please return completed from to the Nurse Manager of Lactation Services.

Lactation Clinical Internship Participant Handbook
Adapted from BSC
7/20/10

Used with Permission Cabarrus College of Health Sciences, Concord, NC

Appendix 6

Documentation Forms

Breastfeeding Observation Form
History Form
Lactation Consultant Chart
Assessment Of Mother And Infant
Milk Intake Worksheet
Sore Nipple History
Slow Weight Gain History

BREASTFEEDING OBSERVATION FORM

Baby's First Name _____ Baby's Age _____ Baby's Birth Weight

Description of nursing situation: _____

Signs the breastfeeding is going well	Signs that there may be problems

GENERAL

Mother:
□ Mother looks healthy
□ Mother is relaxed and comfortable
□ Signs of bonding between mom & baby

Mother:
□ Mother looks exhausted
□ Mother looks depressed or tense
□ Mother doesn't look at the infant or hold it closely

Baby:
□ Baby looks healthy
□ Baby is relaxed and comfortable
□ Baby roots for the breast

Baby:
□ Baby looks thin
□ Baby looks sick or irritable
□ Baby doesn't root or look for the nipple

BREASTS

□ Mother says nipples and breasts are pain free
□ Mother supports breasts while nursing

□ Breasts are red, hard or look sore
□ Nipples/areola are red, cracked or bleeding
□ Mother puts her fingers too close to the nipple

BABY'S POSITION

□ Baby's mouth and body is in alignment with the breast
□ Baby is held close to the mother's body
□ All of the baby's extremities are supported
□ Mother positions her nipple at the height of the baby's nose

□ Baby is laid on his back with his head turned toward the breast
□ Baby appears to be dangling in mother's arms
□ Baby's extremities are not supported
□ Baby's mouth is positioned across or above the nipple

BABY'S ATTACHMENT

□ More areola is seen above the baby's top lip
□ Baby's mouth has a wide gape
□ Lips are flanged out
□ Chin is pushed into the breast and the nose is clear of the breast

□ More of the areola is seen beneath the bottom lip
□ Baby's mouth is not opened wide
□ Lips are sucked in
□ Baby's nose is pushed into the breast and/or there is space between the chin and breast

FEEDING

□ Baby has slow deep sucks
□ Baby pauses, but re-starts sucking without prodding
□ Baby lets go of the breasts when done
□ Nipple is round when released

□ Rapid short sucks, few or no swallows
□ Baby needs prodding to keep sucking
□ Baby never comes off the breast or mother takes him off
□ Nipple is misshapen when release

Adapted from UNICEF/WHO BREASTFEEDING Form © Lactation Education Consultants 2012 – used with permission.

Lactation History

Date_____ Why are you here? _____

Maternal History   Pre-pregnancy weight_____ weight gained _____

How is your overall health _____ Back to work/when_____

Ever had a serious illness anytime in your life? _____ Any skin conditions _____

Depression ____ Meds _____Herbals_____ Birth control_____

Smoker in home_____ Fluids/day_____ Dairy intake _____

Ages of other children in the home_____ Breastfeeding history _____

Family allergies_____ Thyroid tested/why_____ Breast surgery/trauma _____

Infertility/miscarriages_____ Drugs used _____ PCOS _____

Breast changes/size/color_____ Yeast infections/kind and when_____

Parenting/Bf books/classes_____ How long are you planning to breastfeed? _____

Delivery

Length of labor_____ Induction _____ C/Sec_____ Vaginal_____ Forceps/Vacuum_____

Medications in labor_____ Epidural_____ Length_____ Episiotomy_____

Complications_____ Happy with birth_____

Infant History/Hospital

Birth weight_____ D/C weight_____ Other weights _____

Apgars _____ Time of 1st feed/quality_____

Hypoglycemia_____ Formula/bottles/pacifiers given in hospital/why _____

Describe feeds in hospital_____ Jaundice ___ RX _____

Other problems _____ Milk surge/when/describe_____ Engorgement_____

Current History   Age today _____

Pumping/why _____ Kind of pump _____ Nipple soreness/when _____

Number of Feeds/24h_____ Length_____ Breasts 1 2 Who ends feed_____

Void/24h_____ Stools/24h_____ Color_____ Amount of stool _____

Fussy periods_____ Spitting/vomiting _____ Blood in stools _____

Pacifier/why_____ Supplements/kind _____ Amount/24 _____ Given how_____

© Lactation Education Consultants—Used with permission.

The author prints the form with blank space on the right to allow for note taking

LACTATION CONSULTATION CHART

MOTHER_____AGE____OCCUPATION_____

DAD_____AGE____OCCUPATION_____

BABY_____G/P_____BF EXPERIENCE_____

ADDRESS_____PHONE_____

BIRTH DATE_____GEST. AGE_____WEIGHT_____D/C WEIGHT_____

OB/CNM_____HOSPITAL_____BF CLASS_____

TIME OF FIRST BF_____MEDS/ANESTHESIA_____PITOCIN?_____

VACUUM/FORCEPS_____C/S_____VAG___COMPLICATIONS_____

ALLERGIES_____BR. SURGERY/TRAUMA_____THYROID DX____

INFERTILITY_____WT. GAIN IN PREG_____BR. CHANGES_____

MEDICATIONS_____ILLNESS/HX DEPRESSION_____

ABX_____SMOKING_____BREASTFEEDING GOALS_____

E-MAIL ADDRESS_____

HOSPITAL/OFFICE VISIT: (DATE)____   NOTES:

LENGTH OF TIME SINCE BIRTH_____HRS

BREASTFEEDS SINCE BIRTH _____

FORMULA GIVEN SINCE BIRTH _____

REASON_____

hypoglycemia? _____ /When?_____

BREASTS/NIPPLES _____

SPECIFIC MATERNAL/INFANT CONCERNS:

****

EDUCATION PROVIDED: FURTHER NOTES:

____Feeding cues
____Frequency of feeds
____Ascertaining good latch/how to latch
____Positioning
____Laid-back breastfeeding
____Satiation cues/intake-output/normal stooling
____Engorgement relief
____Second Night
____Maternal diet
____Skin to skin
____Gentle waking
____RPS
____Other

ASSESSMENT OF MOTHER AND INFANT

Mother's initials:	Age:	Infant's first name:	Age:

Presenting complaint:

Date of initial consultation:

1. Factors from the history that may be contributing to the problem

2. Describe the feeding, sleeping and output patterns of this infant.

3. What interventions has the mother tried prior to this visit?

Documentation of weight gain/loss since birth	Date	Weight	Amount of loss or gain
Birth weight			
Hospital discharge weight			
Weight at consultation			

Comments:

Physical assessment of the mother

Overall appearance & manner	
Breasts (size, shape, placement of lactiferous ducts, lactation status, abnormalities)	
Nipples (size, graspability, integrity)	

Comments:

Physical assessment of the infant

Hydration/skin turgor	
Skin color	
Muscle tone, activity level	
Oral cavity, frenulum, palate	
Suckle	

Comments:

Feeding Assessment (Use *Breastfeeding Observation Form* and *Milk Intake Worksheet)*

4. What is your assessment of this mother's milk supply?

5. Describe how the baby fed.

    A.   Did you hear audible swallows?

    B.   How long were the baby's eyes open during the feed?

    C.   Did the baby do more nutritive or non-nutritive sucking?

    D.   Did the baby detach from the breast spontaneously?

    E.   How was the baby's demeanor when he was removed from the breast?

6. Do your physical findings suggest that this is primarily an infant problem or a maternal problem? Please explain your answer.

7. Are there any known medical or physical problems of either mother or infant that you believe are impacting on this condition?

8. Were there any interventions or steps in the plan of care that the mother believed she could not comply with or carry out? Please explain your answer.

9. Were there any suggestions you would have liked to make but didn't? Please explain your answer.

10.What is your lactation diagnosis/assessment of this dyad?

MILK INTAKE WORKSHEET (More applicable for infant less than 4 months of age)

Mother's name_____ Date_____

Time breasts were last emptied_____

   ☐ By pumping

   ☐ One breast

   ☐ Two breasts

Time of feeding assessment _____

Time between breasts being emptied and feeding assessment _____

Birth weight_____ lb/oz   Last previous weight_____ lb/oz

Nude weight today_____ lb/oz   _____ grams

Diapered weight (AC) _____ grams   Put to   R   L   breast

PC weight _____ grams   Intake _____ gm/ml   Put to   R   L   breast

PC weight _____ grams   Intake _____ gm/ml   Put to   R   L   breast

PC weight _____ grams   Intake _____ gm/ml   Put to   R   L   breast

PC weight _____ grams   Intake _____ gm/ml

Total intake from breasts (PC - AC weights) =_____gm/ml

Pumped residual: R _____ ml   +   L _____ ml   =   _____ ml total residual

Estimated milk production (EMP) = total intake from the breasts + pumped residual _____ ml

Divide EMP by number of hours since breasts were emptied = _____ Estimated Hourly Production

Estimated Hourly Production X 24 = _____ml or _____oz Theoretical daily production

Estimated milk needs of infant based on: ☐ Birth weight   ☐ Current weight   ☐ Expected weight
(whichever is higher)

Desired weight in total number of ounces _____ ÷ 6 = _____ total number of ounces needed in 24h

Estimated production is: ☐ Under   ☐ Over   estimated needs by _____oz/24h

Nipple Pain Questionnaire

Date_____ Mother's name_____ Baby's name_____
Nipple Size: R diameter_____ R length_____ L diameter_____ L length_____

1. When did you start to have nipple pain?
   ☐ The first time the baby breastfed
   ☐ During the first day at the hospital
   ☐ When my milk supply increased greatly (usually day 3 or 4)
   ☐ Other_____

2. Is the pain on one or both nipples?   ☐ One nipple   ☐ Both nipples

3. Does one nipple hurt more than the other or are both about the same?
   ☐ One nipple hurts more than the other
        If so, on which side?   ☐ Right   ☐ Left
   ☐ Both about the same
   ☐ Fluctuates day to day

4. When does the nipple pain occur?
   ☐ As the baby latches on
   ☐ During the entire feeding
   ☐ Starts out okay, but then hurts more as the feeding goes along
   ☐ Hurts on and off throughout the feeding
   ☐ Hurts after the feeding
   ☐ Hurts at times unrelated to a feeding
   ☐ Hurts all the time

5. Describe the pain.

☐ tugging	☐ aching	☐ biting
☐ tingling	☐ throbbing	☐ stinging
☐ irritating	☐ itching	☐ shooting
☐ rubbing	☐ pinching	☐ burning
☐ scraping	☐ sharp	

6. What is the shape of the nipple when the baby comes off the breast?

☐ normal	☐ creased	☐ pinched
☐ elongated	☐ ridged	☐ like a new lipstick
☐ peaked	☐ pointed	☐ flattened
☐ smashed	☐ stepped on	☐ squished

7. Does your nipple turn white at the end of the feeding?   ☐ Yes   ☐ No

8. Do your nipples turn white at any other time?   ☐ Yes   ☐ No
   Do you have Raynaud's phenomenon?   ☐ Yes   ☐ No
   Do you have a circulation problem?   ☐ Yes   ☐ No

9. Describe if your nipple is a different color from usual.

☐ no change ☐ deep pink ☐ blanched white
☐ lighter than normal ☐ red ☐ has a white stripe
☐ pink ☐ purple

10. Is there any nipple damage? ☐ Yes ☐ No
    If yes, what kind of damage?

☐ abrasion ☐ blister ☐ piece missing
☐ crack ☐ scab ☐ bleeding

11. Where is the nipple pain occurring?　　　　　Draw where you feel the pain.

☐ On the face of the nipple
☐ On the side of the nipple
☐ At the base of the nipple

☐ All over the nipple

☐ On the areola

12. Does it hurt to wear clothing? ☐ All the time ☐ Sometimes ☐ No

13. Are you using a breast pump? ☐ Yes ☐ No
    If yes, does it hurt when you use the pump? ☐ Do not know ☐ Yes ☐ No
    If yes, what brand and type of pump are you using?_____

14. On a scale from zero to ten, if zero is no pain and ten is the most pain you have ever experienced, please mark on the line where you would rate your nipple pain?

0   1   2   3   4   5   6   7   8   9   10

15. Breastfeeding Sensation Scale
    ☐ No sensation
    ☐ Strong pulling and tugging that feels good
    ☐ Strong pulling and tugging that causes no discomfort
    ☐ Strong pulling and tugging that causes some discomfort
    ☐ Pinching that is somewhat uncomfortable
    ☐ Really hurts or feels like biting
    ☐ Unbearable, excruciating pain and had to take baby off

16. What have you been doing to deal with the nipple pain?
    ☐ Applying a topical preparation – If so, what?_____
    ☐ Wearing breast shells
    ☐ Wearing breast pads
    ☐ Taking pain medication – If so, what?_____
    ☐ Stopped breastfeeding – If so, how long ago?_____
    ☐ Pumping and feeding my baby my milk– If so, for how long?_____
    ☐ Putting up with it and waiting for it to get better
    ☐ Suffering through the pain
    ☐ Other_____

17. Do you have a rash anywhere on your body? ☐ Yes ☐ No
    If yes, where?_____

18. Do your nipples itch?   ☐ Yes   ☐ No

19. What do you think is causing your nipple pain?

20. How is your baby doing?

21. Are you now or have you recently taken any medications?   ☐ Yes   ☐ No
     If yes, what?_____

22. Is your baby now or has your baby recently taken any medications?   ☐ Yes   ☐ No
     If yes, what?_____

23. Does your baby have oral thrush?   ☐ Yes   ☐ No

24. Does your baby have a diaper rash?   ☐ Yes   ☐ No

25. Do you wear artificial fingernails?   ☐ Yes   ☐ No

26. Do you wear fingernail polish?   ☐ Yes   ☐ No

27. Do you have long fingernails?   ☐ Yes   ☐ No

28. Are you experiencing breast pain?   ☐ Yes   ☐ No
     If no, you are finished.
     If yes, how would you describe your breast pain?
        ☐ aching all over
        ☐ tingling sensation
        ☐ shooting pain
        ☐ burning pain
        ☐ pain that radiates down my arm
        ☐ pain that radiates around the side to my back

29. Draw where on the breast you are experiencing the pain.

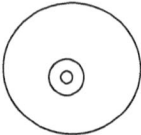 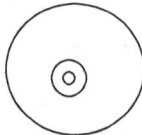

     Right breast   Left breast

30. On a scale from zero to ten, if zero is no pain and ten is the most pain you have ever experienced, please mark on the line where you would rate your breast pain?

0   1   2   3   4   5   6   7   8   9   10

31. When does the breast pain occur?
        ☐ after feedings
        ☐ during feedings
        ☐ all the time
        ☐ at times not related to feedings

Low Weight Gain or Low Milk Supply

Mother's name _____ **Baby's name**_____

Understanding the Process

How is breastfeeding going for you?

Why do you think you do not have enough milk?

What parenting books have you read?

How does your baby let you know he/she wants to feed?

When did your baby feed during the past 24 hours (circle the times)?

     AM: 12 1 2 3 4 5 6 7 8 9 10 11   PM: 12 1 2 3 4 5 6 7 8 9 10 11

How many times in 24 hours does your baby breastfeed? <6 6-7 8-9 10-11 12+

How many times does your baby feed between the hours of 12 midnight and 6 am?

     ☐ One   ☐ Two   ☐ Three   ☐ Four

How long does your baby spend at each feeding? <5 min 6-15 16-25 26-45 >45

Feeding Behavior

Does your baby seem to nurse "all the time"?	☐ Yes	☐ No
Do feedings last an hour or more?	☐ Yes	☐ No
Does your baby end the feeding?	☐ Yes	☐ No
Do you end the feeding?	☐ Yes	☐ No
Does your baby release the first breast before being offered second breast?	☐ Yes	☐ No
Do you alternate the breast on which you start a feeding?	☐ Yes	☐ No
Does your baby suck on a pacifier, thumb/fingers, or parent's finger?	☐ Yes	☐ No
Does your baby prefer one breast?	☐ Yes	☐ No

    If yes, which one?   ☐ Right   ☐ Left   ☐N/A

Does your baby

Feed at both breasts at each feeding?	☐ Sometimes	☐ Usually
Feed at one breast per feeding?	☐ Sometimes	☐ Usually

Describe your baby's behavior at the start of a feeding:

Is your baby eager?	☐ Yes	☐ No
Does your baby cry when offered the breast?	☐ Yes	☐ No
Does the baby fall asleep at the start of the feeding?	☐ Yes	☐ No
Are your baby's eyes closed at the start of the feeding?	☐ Yes	☐ No
Does your baby wake for feedings during the night?	☐ Yes	☐ No
Are you waking the baby for feedings during the day?	☐ Yes	☐ No
Are you limiting your baby's feedings?	☐ Yes	☐ No
Is your baby satisfied after breastfeeding?	☐ Yes	☐ No

Hospital Practices

How many bags of IV fluid did you receive during labor?   None 1 2 3 4 5 6 7 8

How long was your labor? _____ hours   How long was your pushing stage?_____ minutes

Was your baby suctioned after birth?	☐ Yes	☐ No
Did your baby breastfeed during the first hour after birth?	☐ Yes	☐ No
Did you have the baby with you all the time in the hospital?	☐ Yes	☐ No

Did the baby leave your hospital room at any time?	☐ Yes	☐ No
Did your baby receive any formula while in the hospital?	☐ Yes	☐ No
Was your baby jaundiced?	☐ Yes	☐ No
Did your baby have low blood sugar?	☐ Yes	☐ No
Did your baby have any bruising?	☐ Yes	☐ No
Was your baby's clavicle broken?	☐ Yes	☐ No
Was your baby circumcised?	☐ Yes	☐ No
Was your baby subjected to painful or invasive tests in the hospital?	☐ Yes	☐ No
Tests for blood sugar If yes, how many times? ____	☐ Yes	☐ No
Tests for bilirubin If yes, how many times? ____	☐ Yes	☐ No
Other blood tests If yes, how many times? ____	☐ Yes	☐ No
Suctioning If yes, how many times? ____	☐ Yes	☐ No
Other _____ If yes, how many times? ____	☐ Yes	☐ No

Discomfort

Are you in any pain?	☐ Yes	☐ No
Nipples?	☐ Yes	☐ No
Breasts?	☐ Yes	☐ No
Back?	☐ Yes	☐ No
Leg?	☐ Yes	☐ No
Cesarean incision?	☐ Yes	☐ No
Episiotomy?		
Other _____		
Are you having any problems with bowel or bladder control?	☐ Yes	☐ No
Have you had plugged ducts?	☐ Yes	☐ No
Have you had mastitis?	☐ Yes	☐ No

Milk Transfer

When your baby breastfeeds

Do you hear swallowing?	☐ Yes	☐ No
Do you hear loud gulping at the start of the feeding?	☐ Yes	☐ No
Does your baby choke?	☐ Yes	☐ No
Does your baby pull off the breast?	☐ Yes	☐ No
Do you see milk squirting from your breasts when baby lets go?	☐ Yes	☐ No
Are you using a nipple shield?	☐ Yes	☐ No
If yes, are you pumping your breasts after each feeding?	☐ Yes	☐ No

Activity Level

How many children under five years are you caring for?
    ☐One   ☐Two   ☐Three   ☐Four

How many animals are you caring for?
    ☐Zero   ☐One   ☐Two   ☐Three   ☐Four

Are you caring for any extended family members?	☐ Yes	☐ No
Are you caring for a sick relative or friend?	☐ Yes	☐ No
Do you have other care giving responsibilities?	☐ Yes	☐ No
Are you so busy that you feed your baby less often?	☐ Yes	☐ No
Are you so busy you need help taking care of your baby?	☐ Yes	☐ No
Do you feel as if you are under too much stress?	☐ Yes	☐ No
Are you getting enough sleep?	☐ Yes	☐ No
Are you tired?	☐ Yes	☐ No
Are you able to sleep when there is an opportunity to sleep?	☐ Yes	☐ No
When do you usually take a nap each day? _____		
Do you have enough help with household chores?	☐ Yes	☐ No
Do you have family and friends who have been helping you?	☐ Yes	☐ No

Nutrition

Did you have an eating disorder as a teenager?	☐ Yes	☐ No
Do you severely restrict any foods from your diet?	☐ Yes	☐ No
Do you currently have an eating disorder?	☐ Yes	☐ No
Are you on any special kind of a diet?	☐ Yes	☐ No
Are you a vegan?	☐ Yes	☐ No
Have you had gastric bypass surgery?	☐ Yes	☐ No

How much water do you drink daily? _____

How much vitamin B6 do you consume daily?* _____

* Consumption should be less than 25 mg/d; 600mg/d have decreased milk in some women.

Psychological

Does your family support your wish to breastfeed your baby?	☐ Yes	☐ No
Do you feel pressured to breastfeed?	☐ Yes	☐ No
Do you feel depressed?	☐ Yes	☐ No
Do you like being a mother?	☐ Yes	☐ No
Is motherhood anything like what you thought it would be?	☐ Yes	☐ No
Are you enjoying breastfeeding?	☐ Yes	☐ No
Was this a planned pregnancy?	☐ Yes	☐ No

When did you get your first period and was it regular? _____

Have you ever been diagnosed with anorexia or bulimia? ☐ Yes ☐ No

Chemical Exposure

Are you eating, drinking or chewing sage, parsley, peppermint?	☐ Yes	☐ No
Were you treated with steroids to help your baby's lungs develop?	☐ Yes	☐ No
Were you on an SSRI (depression medication) during your pregnancy?	☐ Yes	☐ No
Were you raised in a farming community?	☐ Yes	☐ No
Was your mother raised in a farming community?	☐ Yes	☐ No

How many cigarettes do you smoke daily? ☐Zero ☐Five ☐Ten ☐More _____

When was the last time you used a recreational drug? _____

Have you had any exposure to toxic chemicals? ☐ Yes ☐ No

What medications are you taking now? _____

What medications were you taking before you became pregnant? _____

What medications did you take during this pregnancy? _____

Nipple Appearance

Unusual appearance of the nipple:

At rest	With compression
☐ evert	☐ evert
☐ flat	☐ flat
☐ dimpled	☐ dimpled
☐ inverted	☐ inverted
	☐ retracting

Have you ever had nipple surgery? ☐ Yes ☐ No

Have you ever had a nipple ring? ☐ Yes ☐ No

Nipple Size

Right nipple diameter _____ Left nipple diameter _____

Right nipple length _____ Left nipple length _____

Nipple compressible: ☐soft ☐firm ☐meaty

Breast History

Have you had any breast surgery?		☐ Yes	☐ No
Augmentation?	☐ Yes ☐ No	If yes, date: _____	
Implants?	☐ Yes ☐ No	If yes, date: _____	
Reduction?	☐ Yes ☐ No	If yes, date: _____	
Cysts removal?	☐ Yes ☐ No	If yes, date: _____	
Biopsy?	☐ Yes ☐ No	If yes, date: _____	
Change in nipple sensitivity?		☐ Yes	☐ No
Chest tube as a premature baby?		☐ Yes	☐ No
Have you ever had any trauma to your breasts?		☐ Yes	☐ No
Have you ever had bruises on your breasts?		☐ Yes	☐ No
Have you ever had radiation to your breasts? *		☐ Yes	☐ No
Did you have repeated x-rays/imaging of your chest area as a child?		☐ Yes	☐ No
Have your experienced any burns on your breasts?		☐ Yes	☐ No
Have you had breast cancer?		☐ Yes	☐ No
Have you ever had non-lactation mastitis? **		☐ Yes	☐ No

* Per Dow K.H., et al., (1994): 34% of women can lactate after radiation treatment.
** Per James Racinski, MD. (2000 conference); NY: It could be hard to initiate lactation.

Breast Assessment

☐ asymmetry   ☐ conical/tubular   ☐ hypoplasia (underdeveloped)

Distance between breasts _____

Breast texture: ☐   elastic   ☐   firm

Bra cup size   before pregnancy_____   during pregnancy_____   now_____

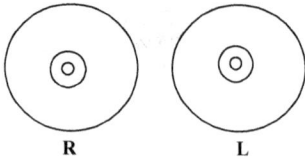

Draw in surgical scars or other anomalies.

R   L

Do you feel your milk "let-down?"	☐ Yes	☐ No
Do your breasts leak?	☐ Yes	☐ No
Did your breasts enlarge during your pregnancy?	☐ Yes	☐ No
Did you feel your milk "come-in" after the birth of the baby?	☐ Yes	☐ No
If yes, what day? _____		
Did you experience extreme engorgement?	☐ Yes	☐ No
If yes, how long did it last?_____		
Was your labor induced?	☐ Yes	☐ No

Medications

Did you receive any medications for labor, delivery, or postpartum?

Magnesium sulfate	☐ Yes	☐ No
Antibiotic	☐ Yes	☐ No
Pitocin	☐ Yes	☐ No
Epidural	☐ Yes	☐ No
Pain reliever	☐ Yes	☐ No
Stool softener	☐ Yes	☐ No
Do you have a prescription for birth control?	☐ Yes	☐ No
Are you using any kind of birth control now?	☐ Yes	☐ No
DepoProvera	☐ Yes	☐ No
Progestin only (Micronor)	☐ Yes	☐ No
Combination progestin/estrogen pills	☐ Yes	☐ No
Combination progestin/estrogen patch	☐ Yes	☐ No

Combination progestin/estrogen nuva-ring	☐ Yes	☐ No
Combination progestin/estrogen IUD Mirena (levonorgestrel)	☐ Yes	☐ No
Combination progestin/estrogen IUD paraguard	☐ Yes	☐ No
Other_____	☐ Yes	☐ No
Are you experiencing heavy vaginal bleeding?	☐ Yes	☐ No

Medical Conditions

Did any previous babies have problems gaining weight?	☐N/A	☐ Yes	☐ No
Do you have any infections?		☐ Yes	☐ No
Are you anemic?		☐ Yes	☐ No

Do you have

Diabetes	☐ Yes	☐ No
If yes, what kind? ☐gestational ☐type I ☐type II		
Allergies	☐ Yes	☐ No
Lupus	☐ Yes	☐ No
Parkinson Disease	☐ Yes	☐ No
Did you have major bleeding after the birth?	☐ Yes	☐ No
Were you given a blood transfusion?	☐ Yes	☐ No
Was your labor stressful for you?	☐ Yes	☐ No
Have you ever had radiation to your brain?	☐ Yes	☐ No
Do you have high blood pressure?	☐ Yes	☐ No
Did you have high blood pressure before you became pregnant?	☐ Yes	☐ No
Did it develop into preeclampsia during the pregnancy?	☐ Yes	☐ No
Pregnancy induced hypertention?	☐ Yes	☐ No
HELLP syndrome (variant or complication of pre-eclampsia)?	☐ Yes	☐ No
Where your legs swollen?	☐ Yes	☐ No
If yes, for how long? _____		
Does a family member have a history of high blood pressure?	☐ Yes	☐ No
If yes, what relation? _____		

Have you ever had or been diagnosed with

Hypothyroidism	☐ Yes	☐ No
Hyperthyroidism	☐ Yes	☐ No
Thyroid surgery?	☐ Yes	☐ No
Pituitary tumor	☐ Yes	☐ No
Sjögren's syndrome	☐ Yes	☐ No
Do you have any other medical problems?	☐ Yes	☐ No
If yes, what? _____		

Hormone Balance

Are you pregnant?	☐ Yes	☐ No
Did you have problems getting pregnant	☐ Yes	☐ No
Did you have irregular periods?	☐ Yes	☐ No
Were you on birth control pills as a teenager?	☐ Yes	☐ No
Was this an in vitro fertilization?	☐ Yes	☐ No
Are you using a hormone patch for postpartum depression?	☐ Yes	☐ No
Have you taken emergency contraception?	☐ Yes	☐ No
Is there a history in your family of lack of progesterone?	☐ Yes	☐ No
Is there a history in your family of lack of prolactin?	☐ Yes	☐ No
Did a sister have difficulties with breastfeeding?	☐ Yes	☐ No
Did your mother or aunts have difficulties with breastfeeding?	☐ Yes	☐ No
Do you have Congenital Adrenal Hyperplasia?	☐ Yes	☐ No
Have you been told you have cysts on your ovaries?	☐ Yes	☐ No
Do you have polycystic ovarian syndrome?	☐ Yes	☐ No
Do you have elevated cholesterol?	☐ Yes	☐ No

Have your breasts leaked when not pregnant or breastfeeding? ☐ Yes ☐ No
Do you have brown velvety patches on your skin? ☐ Yes ☐ No
Do you have endometriosis? ☐ Yes ☐ No
During your pregnancy did you notice
    Abdominal or facial hair growth? ☐ Yes ☐ No
    Pimples on your face, chest, or back? ☐ Yes ☐ No
    Balding? ☐ Yes ☐ No
    Deepening of your voice? ☐ Yes ☐ No
    Enlarged clitoris? ☐ Yes ☐ No
    Development of skin tags (A sign of insulin resistance)? ☐ Yes ☐ No
Do you have
    Insulin resistance ☐ Yes ☐ No
    Elevated LH:FSH>2 ☐ Yes ☐ No
    Elevated estrogen ☐ Yes ☐ No

Your height _____   Your current weight _____

Your weight before pregnancy _____   Your weight at end of pregnancy _____

Did you have a rapid weight loss in the early postpartum? _____ (Sign of thyroiditis)

Your Baby

What color is the baby's urine?
    ☐ Clear ☐ Yellow ☐ Bright yellow ☐ Orange ☐ Red
How many wet diapers does your baby have in 24 hours?
    ☐ 1-2 ☐ 3-4 ☐ 5-6 ☐ 7-8 ☐ 9 or more
What color are your baby's bowel movements?
    ☐ black ☐ green ☐ yellow ☐ yellowish-brown ☐ brown
How many times in 24 hours does your baby have a bowel movement?
    ☐ 1-2 ☐ 3-4 ☐ 5-6 ☐ 7-8 ☐ 9 or more
What makes you think your baby is not getting enough?
Is the baby receiving any formula now? ☐ Yes ☐ No
How much in 24 hours? _____
Does your baby have reflux? ☐ Yes ☐ No
Was your baby premature? ☐ Yes ☐ No
    If so, how many weeks gestation? _____
Does your baby have any health problems? ☐ Yes ☐ No
    ☐ physical anomalies such as a heart problem, congenital abnormalities
    ☐ central nervous system insult
    ☐ neuromuscular disease such as CP
    ☐ genetic impairment
    ☐ congenital adrenal hyperplasia
    ☐ Down Syndrome
    ☐ hypertonic
    ☐ hypotonic
    Other _____
Is your baby on any medications? ☐ Yes ☐ No
    If yes, what? _____
Was the birth traumatic? ☐ Yes ☐ No
Was your baby's birth assisted with a vacuum? ☐ Yes ☐ No
Was your baby's birth assisted with forceps? ☐ Yes ☐ No
Was the cord wrapped around your baby's neck? ☐ Yes ☐ No
Was your baby suctioned for meconium? ☐ Yes ☐ No

Date of birth_____ Birth weight_____ Discharge weight_____ Current weight_____
Other weights in hospital_____

Physical Assessment

Is this assessment normal?

Palate	☐ Yes	☐ No
Uvula	☐ Yes	☐ No
Lips	☐ Yes	☐ No
Philtrum	☐ Yes	☐ No
Tongue	☐ Yes	☐ No
Frenulum	☐ Yes	☐ No
Chin receding	☐ Yes	☐ No
Nostrils	☐ Yes	☐ No
Breathing	☐ Yes	☐ No
Congested sounding?	☐ Yes	☐ No
Stridor?	☐ Yes	☐ No
Cheeks	☐ Yes	☐ No
Mouth	☐ Yes	☐ No
Gums	☐ Yes	☐ No

Behavioral Assessment

Baby appears in pain	☐ Yes	☐ No
Turns head to only one side	☐ Yes	☐ No
Sleepy	☐ Yes	☐ No
Rooting	☐ Yes	☐ No
Noisy home	☐ Yes	☐ No
Offensive smells in the home	☐ Yes	☐ No
Breast aversion	☐ Yes	☐ No
Does your baby have allergies?	☐ Yes	☐ No
Does your baby have pyloric stenosis	☐ Yes	☐ No
Have allergy tests been run on your baby?	☐ Yes	☐ No

Sucking

Evaluation of the baby's suck by IBCLC	☐ Strong	☐ OK	☐ Weak
Evaluation of the baby's suck by mother	☐ Strong	☐ OK	☐ Weak

How does it feel when your baby is sucking on your breast?

Tugging or pulling	☐ Yes	☐ No
Pinching or biting	☐ Yes	☐ No
Like the breast pump	☐ Yes	☐ No

Observation of a Feeding

Mother is in a comfortable position	☐ Yes	☐ No
Baby is in a comfortable position	☐ Yes	☐ No
Baby sustains 10 or more sucks in a row at the start of the feeding	☐ Yes	☐ No
Pauses are less than 10 seconds at the start of the feeding	☐ Yes	☐ No
Angle at the corner of the baby's mouth is over 130 degrees	☐ Yes	☐ No
Mother appears tense	☐ Yes	☐ No
Mother's hand is on baby's head	☐ Yes	☐ No
Baby's eyes are closed at the start of the feeding (over 1 week old)	☐ Yes	☐ No
Baby pulls in the lips	☐ Yes	☐ No
Baby's cheeks are dimpling	☐ Yes	☐ No
Baby makes clicking sounds (i.e., releases suction)	☐ Yes	☐ No
Milk leaks out of the corner of the baby's mouth	☐ Yes	☐ No

Appendix 7

Relevant Professional Organizations

INTERNATIONAL BOARD OF LACTATION CONSULTANT EXAMINERS (IBLCE)

6402 Arlington Boulevard, Suite 350

Falls Church, VA 22042, USA

Phone: +1 703-560-7330

Fax: +1 703-560-7332

Email: international@iblce.org

www.iblce.org

INTERNATIONAL LACTATION CONSULTANT ASSOCIATION (ILCA)

2501 Aerial Center Parkway, Suite 103

Morrisville, North Carolina, 27560, USA

Phone: +1 919-861-5577

Toll Free 1-888-ILCA-IS-U (452-2478)

Fax: +1 919-459-2075

E-mail: info@ilca.org

www.ilca.org

LACTATION EDUCATION ACCREDITATION AND APPROVAL REVIEW COMMITTEE (LEAARC)

2501 Aerial Center Parkway, Suite 103

Morrisville, North Carolina, 27560, USA

Phone: +1 919-459-6106

Fax: +1 919-459-2075

Email: info@leaarc.org

www.leaarc.org

References

Andersen, P.A. (2004). *The complete idiot's guide to body language.* New York, NY: Penguin Group.

Bannister, S.L., Raszka, Jr., W.V., & Maloney, C.G. (2010). What makes a great clinical teacher in pediatrics? Lessons learned from the literature. *Pediatrics, 125,* 863-865. doi: 10.1542/peds.2010-0628.

Barger , J. (2002). Acquiring the LC role: A theoretical perspective. Clinical instructor workshop at ILCA Conference, Boca Raton FL. (Also in Lauwers, J. & Swisher, A. (2011). *Counseling the nursing mother* (5th ed.). Sudbury, MA: Jones & Bartlett. pp 637-39.)

Benner, P. (1984). *From novice to expert: Excellence and power in clinical nursing practice.* Menlo Park, CA: Addison-Wesley.

Birthingway College of Midwifery. (2012). Lactation Consultant Pathway 2. Retrieved from http://www.birthingway.edu/program-info/breastfeeding-counselor-and-lactation-consultant-programs/lactation-consultant-pathway-2.htm.

Brainy Quote. (2012). Retrieved from http://www.brainyquote.com/quotes/quotes/s/samueltayl156374.html.

Buchel, T.L., & Edwards, F.D. (2005). Characteristics of effective clinical instructors. *Family Medicine, 31*(1), 30-35.

Burrows, D.E. (1995). The nurse teacher's role in the promotion of reflective practice. *Nurse Education Today, 15,* 346-350.

CAAHEP (Commission on Accreditation of Allied Health Education Programs). (2011). Standards and guidelines for the accreditation of lactation education programs. Retrieved from http://leaarc.org/download/LEAARC_StandardsGuidelines.pdf.

Carnegie, D. (1936). *How to win friends and influence people.* New York, NY: Simon & Schuster.

Carolinas Medical Center-NorthEast Women's and Children's Services/Cabarrus College Lactation Clinical Internship. (2012). Retrieved from http://www.cabarruscollege.edu/programs/continuing_education/lactation/lactation.cfm.

College Board. (2012). College-level examination program. Retrieved from http://clep.collegeboard.org/.

DSST. (2012). DANTES Subject standardized tests. Retrieved from http://www.getcollegecredit.com/.

ELCA. (2012). The Egyptian Lactation Consultants' Association. Retrieved from http://elcaonline.net/portal/Activities/EducationalWork/tabid/445/Default.aspx.

Gibson, J. (2009). The five "Es" of an excellent teacher. *The Clinical Teacher, 6,* 3-8.

Goertzen, J., Stewart, M., & Weston, W. (1995). Effective teaching behaviors of rural family medicine preceptors. *Canadian Medical Association Journal, 153,* 161-168.

Grasha, A.F. (1994). A matter of style: The teacher as expert, formal authority, personal model, facilitator, and delegator. *College Teaching, 42,* 142-149.

Grasha, A. & Riechmann, S. (2012). Teaching style survey. Retrieved from http://www.longleaf.net/teachingstyle.html.

Hagen, S. (2008). *The everything body language book*. Avon, MA: Adams Media, division of F+W Media, Inc.

HRSA (Health Resources and Services Administration). (2012). *Telehealth*. Retrieved from http://www.hrsa.gov/ruralhealth/about/telehealth/.

IBLCE (International Board of Lactation Consultant Examiners). (2010). *Clinical competencies for the practice of International Board Certified Lactation Consultants (IBCLCs)*. Retrieved from http://www.iblce.org/upload/downloads/ClinicalCompetencies.pdf.

IBLCE (International Board of Lactation Consultant Examiners). (2012). *Certification*. Retrieved from http://www.iblce.org/certification.

IBLCE (International Board of Lactation Consultant Examiners). (2011a) *General education guidelines*. Retrieved from http://iblce.org/upload/downloads/GeneralEducationGuidelines.pdf.

IBLCE (International Board of Lactation Consultant Examiners). (2011b). *Code of professional conduct for IBCLCs*. Retrieved from http://www.iblce.org/upload/downloads/CodeOfProfessionalConduct.pdf.

IBLCE (International Board of Lactation Consultant Examiners). (2011c). *Pathway 3 plan approval guide for the development and approval of Pathway 3 clinical apprenticeships*. Retrieved from http://www.iblce.org/upload/downloads/Pathway3PlanGuide.pdf.

ILCA (International Lactation Consultant Association). (2012a). *Clinical instruction directory*. Retrieved from http://www.ilca.org/i4a/pages/index.cfm?pageid=3896.

ILCA (International Lactation Consultant Association). (2012b). Lactation matters: Official blog of the International Lactation Consultant Association. Retrieved from http://lactationmatters.org/.

ILCA (International Lactation Consultant Association). (2006). *Standards of practice for International Board Certified Lactation Consultants*. Retrieved from http://www.ilca.org/files/resources/Standards-of-Practice-web.pdf.

IOM (Institute of Medicine), Committee on Quality of Health Care in America. (2001). *Crossing the quality chasm: A new health system for the 21st century*. Washington, DC: The National Academies Press.

Irby, D.M. (1995). Teaching and learning in ambulatory care settings: A thematic review of the literature. *Academic Medicine, 70*, 898-931.

Kassirer, J.P. (2010). Teaching clinical reasoning: Case-based and coached. *Academic Medicine, 85*, 1118-1124.

Kolb, D. (1984). *Experiential learning: Experience as the source of learning and development*. Retrieved from http://www.learning-theories.com/experiential-learning-kolb.html.

Kuhnke, E. (2007). *Body language for dummies*. West Sussex. England: John Wiley & Sons, Ltd.

Kutner, L.A. & Barger, J. (2010). *Clinical experience in lactation: A blueprint for internship* (3rd ed.). Wheaton, IL: Lactation Education Consultants.

Lactation Education Resources. (2012). Online Lactation Consultant Training Program. Retrieved from http://www.leron-line.com/LC_Training_online/Lactation_Consultant_Training_online.htm?gclid=CKuNrK6nwa8CFWkQNAodKC31xg.

LACTNET. (2012). *Lactation information and discussion*. Retrieved from http://www. lsoft.com/scripts/wl.exe?SL1=LACTNET&H=COMMUNITY.LSOFT.COM.

Lambert, D. (2008). *Body language 101*. London, England: Diagram Visual Information, Limited.

Lauwers, J. & Swisher, A. (2011). *Counseling the nursing mother: A lactation consultant's guide*. Sudbury, MA: Jones and Bartlett Learning.

Lawrence, G. (1991). *People types and tiger stripes: A practical guide to learning styles* (3rd ed.). Gainsville, FL: Center for Applications of Psychological Type, Inc.

Lindberg, I., Ohrling, K., & Christensson, K. (2007). Midwives' experience of using videoconferencing to support parents who were discharged early after birth. *Journal of Telemedicine & Telecare, 13*, 202-205.

Masunaga, H. & Hitchock, M.A. (2010). Residents' and faculty's beliefs about the ideal clinical instructor. *Family Medicine, 42*(2), 116-120.

McCarthy, B. & McCarthy D. (2005). *Teaching around the 4MAT cycle: Designing instruction for diverse learners with diverse learning styles*. Thousand Oaks, CA: Corwin Press.

McCarthy, B. & O'Neill-Blackwell, J. (2007). *Hold on, you lost me! Use learning styles to create training that sticks*. Alexandria, VA: American Society for Training and Development.

Millikin University. (2006). *Preceptor roles and responsibilities*. Decatur, IL: Millikin University.

Pennsylvania Resource Organization for Lactation Consultants. (2012). *How to become a lactation consultant*. Retrieved from http://www.pro-lc.org/mentoring_consortium.html.

Presbyterian Hospital. (2012). Lactation Clinical Internship. Retrieved from http:// www.presbyterian.org/site/our_services/womens_services/maternity_services/ the_nursing_mothers_place/internships/.

RGCP (Royal College of General Practioners). (2012). *Workplace based assessment*. Retrieved from http://www.rcgp-curriculum.org.uk/nmrcgp/wpba.aspx.

Rojjanasrirat, W., Wambach, K., & Nelson, E. (in press). A pilot study of home-based videoconferencing for breastfeeding support. *Journal of Human Lactation*.

Ruthman, J., Jackson, J., Cluskey, M.,Flannigan, P., Folse, V.N. & Bunten, J. (2004). Using clinical journaling to capture critical thinking across the curriculum. *Nursing Education Perspectives, 25*, 120-123.

Simkin, P. & Klaus, P. (2004). *When survivors give birth*. Seattle, WA: Classic Day Publishing.

Sutkin, G., Wagner, E., Harris, I. & Schiffer, R. (2008). What makes a good clinical instructor in medicine? A review of the literature. *Academic Medicine, 83*, 452-466.

Truscott, A. (2010). A method of teaching clinical problem-solving skills to primary health care student nurses. *South African Family Practice, 52*, 60-63.

Turpin, G. & Wheeler, S. (2011). *IAPT supervision guidance*. Retrieved from http:// www.iapt.nhs.uk/silo/files/iapt-supervision-guidance-revised-march-2011.pdf.

Union Institute & University. (2012). *Maternal child health: Lactation consulting curriculum*. http://www.myunion.edu/academics/bachelor-of-science/maternal-child-health/curriculum.html.

University of California-San Diego. (2012). *Lactation consultant certificate*. http://extension.ucsd.edu/programs/index.cfm?vAction=certDetail&vCertificateID=104&vStudyAreaID=12.

University of North Carolina at Chapel Hill. (2012). *Carolina Global Breastfeeding Institute: Mary Rose Tully training initiative*. Retrieved from http://cgbi.sph.unc.edu/academics/education/mrtti.

USDA Office of Research and Analysis. (2011). Special supplemental nutrition program For women, infants, and children (WIC) eligibles and coverage – 2000 To 2009: National and state level estimates of the population of women, infants, and children eligible for WIC benefits, Executive summary. Retrieved from http://www.fns.usda.gov/ora/MENU/Published/WIC/FILES/WICEligibles2000-2009Summary.pdf.

Wagner, S., Keane, S., McLeod, B., Bishop, M. (2008). A report: clinical supervision for allied health professionals in rural NSW. Retrieved from http://www.ruralceti.health.nsw.gov.au/.

WHO (World Health Organization). (1981). *International code of marketing of breast-milk substitutes*. Retrieved from http://www.who.int/nutrition/publications/code_english.pdf.

Index

About the Authors

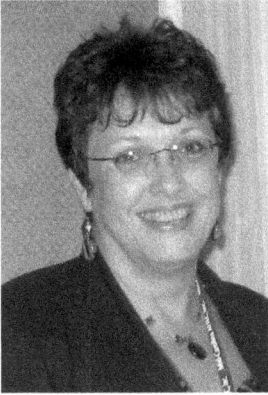

Phyllis Kombol, RN, MSN, IBCLC has been an IBCLC since 1993 and has provided internships for aspiring and new lactation consultants at various worksites for many years. In her current worksite, she is the primary lactation consultant in a tertiary NICU and is part of a team of IBCLCs providing comprehensive lactation services. She has been instrumental in the development of a formalized Lactation Clinical Internship program, which is a collaboration of Carolinas Medical Center-NorthEast and Cabarrus College of Health Sciences Continuing Education Department (see www.Cabarruscollege. edu) in North Carolina, USA. Phyllis is an RN certified in NICU nursing, Clinical Nurse Specialist in Parent-Child Nursing, and has served as adjunct faculty for baccalaureate and master's degree nursing students. She teaches via webinars and conferences several times each year, and is an active member of nursing and lactation professional organizations, as well as Toastmasters International. Phyllis is currently a member of a Clinical Instructor Task Force, working in collaboration with ILCA's Education Committee.

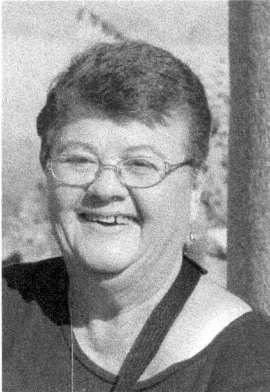

Linda Kutner, BSN, IBCLC, FILCA has worked in the pediatric and lactation field since 1967. She is currently a lactation consultant at Lake Norman Regional Medical Center in North Carolina, USA, seeing both inpatients and outpatients. Linda had an extensive private practice for many years and has worked with some very challenging cases. As well as being a member of AWHONN, she is a charter member of ILCA, and their first U.S. Delegate. She was the 1992-94 ILCA Board of Directors President and served on the IBLCE Board of Directors from 1994-1996. Linda is the primary author of *Clinical Experience in Lactation: A Blueprint for Internship* and was the coordinator for the IBLCE/BSC research project, which ultimately led to IBLCE's Pathway 3 (formerly Pathway F). She currently supervises lactation consultant interns at Lake Norman and serves on the Clinical Instructor Task Force for ILCA. Linda has been a Director and primary lecturer with Lactation Education Consultants since 1995.

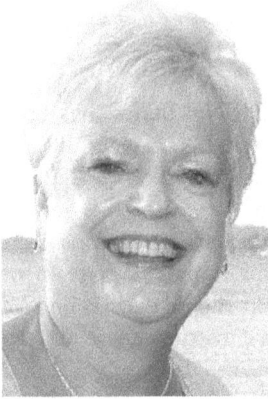

Jan Barger, RN, MA, IBCLC, FILCA is an obstetrical nurse by background and has worked in every aspect of maternal-child health, except the NICU. She taught obstetrics in a school of nursing, providing both didactic and clinical instruction. After becoming a lactation consultant, she has had a private practice, worked with obstetrician/nurse midwife and pediatric groups, and taught a clinical rotation with lactation interns at the University of Chicago Hospital. She co-developed the original ILCA Clinical Instructor Workshop and co-authored *Clinical Experience in Lactation: A Blueprint for Internship.* Jan was the 1990-1992 ILCA President, served on the IBLCE board from 1992-1994, and among other appointments is currently co-chair of the Clinical Instructor Task Force. She has been a director and lecturer with Breastfeeding Support Consultants and Lactation Education Consultants since 1995, as well as teaching about breastfeeding to health professionals in other venues nationally and internationally.

Note: *Clinical Experience in Lactation: A Blueprint for Internship* can be obtained from the ILCA bookstore.